THE *Skinny* SOUP MAKER
RECIPE BOOK

DELICIOUS LOW CALORIE, HEALTHY AND SIMPLE SOUP RECIPES UNDER 100, 200 AND 300 CALORIES. PERFECT FOR ANY DIET AND WEIGHT LOSS PLAN.

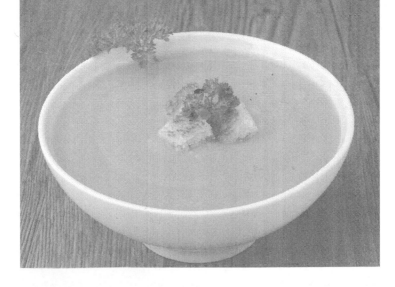

The Skinny Soup Maker Recipe Book.
Delicious Low Calorie, Healthy and Simple Soup Machine Recipes Under 100, 200 and 300 Calories. Perfect For Any Diet and Weight Loss Plan.

A Bell & Mackenzie Publication
First published in 2013 by Bell & Mackenzie Publishing
Copyright © Bell & Mackenzie Publishing 2013

A catalogue record of this book is available from the British Library.

ISBN 978-1-909855-02-1

Disclaimer
The information and advice in this book is intended as a guide only. Any individual should independently seek the advice of a health professional before embarking on a diet. Some recipes may contain nuts or traces of nuts. Those suffering from any allergies associated with nuts should avoid any recipes containing nuts or nut based oils.

Contents

Contents

Contents

Contents

THE Skinny SOUP MAKER RECIPE BOOK

Introduction

Introduction

Soup – a wonderfully versatile, diverse and healthy dish with a multitude of different flavours and inspirations from around the world. The perfect meal, side dish or snack all year round - from the sweet flavours and crunch of spring vegetables to light summery day bisques through to hearty winter broths. Soup can be enjoyed whatever the time of year and with healthy fresh ingredients it's a winner for a balanced diet and can be instrumental in helping you lose weight or maintain your figure without compromising on flavour, taste or leaving you feeling hungry.

Soup is incredibly easy to prepare, economical, low in calories, makes use of whatever leftovers you have in the kitchen and can be frozen. Our skinny soup recipes can help you lose weight because all fall under 100, 200 and 300 calories per serving and most can be prepared and cooked using a soup maker in under 30 minutes.

If you are looking for some new ideas for soup making to help you lose weight, control your diet or to serve up a healthy balanced dish for your family then you will find inspiration here.

The recipes in this book are all written for use with a soup maker but can also be used if you prefer the more traditional stove-top method of soup making.

We hope you enjoy this collection of skinny soups.

What Is A Skinny Soup?

Simply put a 'skinny' soup is one of our delicious soup recipes each falling below either 100, 200 or 300 calories per serving. By calculating the number of calories for each dish we've made it easy for you to count your daily calorie intake as part of a controlled diet or a balanced healthy eating plan.

What This Book Will Do For You

The recipes in this book are all low calorie dishes which make it easy for you to control your overall daily calorie intake. The recommended daily calories are 2000 for women and 2500 for men. Broadly speaking, by consuming this level of calories each day you should maintain your current weight. Reducing the number of calories (a calorie deficit) will result in losing weight. This happens because the body begins to use fat stores for energy to make up the reduction in calories, which in turn results in weight loss. Preparing a number of balanced meals throughout the day and counting each calorie however can be difficult, that's why our skinny soups are so great. We have already counted the calories for each dish making it easy for you to fit this into to your daily eating plan whether you are looking to lose weight, maintain your current figure or are just looking for some great-tasting soup ideas.

I'm Already On A Diet. Can I Use These Recipes?

Yes of course. All the recipes can be great accompaniments to many of the popular calorie-counting diets. We all know that sometimes dieting can result in hunger pangs, cravings and boredom from eating the same old foods day in and day out. Skinny soups can break that cycle by providing filling 'meals in one' which will satisfy you for hours afterwards.

I Am Only Cooking For One. Will This Book Work For Me?

Yes. To make the best use of each dish we have made all servings for four people. Remember you can always refrigerate or freeze portions for another day if you are just cooking for one.

Soup Is Just For Cold Winter Nights Right?

Wrong! While there is nothing better than a bowl of comforting steaming hot broth on a miserable winter's day, soup isn't just for dark cold nights. It can be a vibrant and refreshing alternative on the brightest and hottest of days, and make use of the best seasonal ingredients all year round. Did you know that some soups can also be served chilled? What could be better on a summer's day? Soups can be a wonderful revelation to your day, waking up your taste buds to new possibilities. Think Thai, Chicken & Coconut or Japanese Ramen Noodle Soup and suddenly you have opened yourself up to a world of soup possibilities.

What Makes A Great Soup?

Thankfully you don't have to be a great chef to make an incredible soup and using a soup maker just makes everything even easier. There are however a few key elements to making a great soup.

The Base:
The start to most soups requires a few vegetables to give your soup a rounded flavour. Onions, carrots and celery are a great start.

Stock:
A good quality stock will make the world of difference to the quality of your soup. Use either vegetable, fish or meat stock and if you can make these at home, all the better. You can follow these simple instructions to make homemade stock. If you opt for store-bought stock try to choose a good quality product that is not high in sodium.

Ingredients:
Soup is so versatile that almost any ingredient can be used - whether you are looking for a meaty protein packed dish, an Asian seafood soup, or a thick vegetarian broth using beans and pulses. Certain ingredients will change the consistency of your soup too, for example potatoes and lentils will thicken, while adding some single cream will make it smoother.

Seasoning:
Most soups will require some seasoning. Be careful when choosing your stock that it is not overly high in its sodium content. There are also many popular herbs that compliment soups such as marjoram, thyme, parsley, sage, rosemary, oregano and of course salt and pepper. You should also feel free to experiment. For example: Garlic, ginger and coriander can work well in Asian soups while cumin, turmeric or garam masala can give an authentic Indian feel to your dish.

Garnish:

There is nothing better than serving a homemade soup with a little garnish, which not only looks the part but also adds an extra taste. Depending on your dish, freshly chopped herbs, croutons, a little cream, crème fraiche or freshly grated parmesan are all great finishing touches.

Which Soup Maker?

If you are reading this you will no doubt already have purchased a soup maker. For those who have not, or are considering replacing their appliance there are a few basic considerations when purchasing a soup maker.

Model:

There are 2 main styles of soup maker on the market at the moment. One resembles a traditional blender in appearance and the other a jug-style which looks a little like a modern kettle. The blender style is generally more expensive but offers more flexibility enabling you to brown-off base ingredients for example as well as adjust cooking times. This style also allows you to use the unit as a traditional blender for crushing ice, making smoothies etc. The glass jar also allows you to see the contents as they cook.

The jug/kettle style differs to the blender style by having the blades and motor in the lid of the appliance rather than the base. These units do not have a glass jar so you cannot see the contents while cooking therefore it is necessary to check fill levels to avoid over-filling.

There is no option to brown ingredients with this type of machine and you cannot use raw meat or fish - only cooked. This type of soup maker is very easy to use with pre-programmed settings.

Size:
Soup makers have different capacities depending on the quantity of soup you need to make. They generally range from 1.0 to 1.7 litres. Make your choice of capacity dependant on your needs but remember that you can freeze soup so any extras can be used for another meal.

Power:
This will determine how powerful the appliance will chop and blend. Generally a more powerful motor may see better results but not always! Also a more powerful machine may heat up your soup quicker.

Settings:
There should be multiple heating settings. Usually low, medium, high and simmer. Depending which model you have (blender style or jug/kettle style) you will also have a timer or pre-programmed settings.

Non-stick Heating Plate:
Most appliances will advertise this as a feature. You will no doubt know from your own experience that the ingredients can sometimes stick and can be stubborn to remove afterwards. Make sure you carefully read reviews of the product before purchasing and follow manufacturer's guidelines for use.

Stir Function:

This is a handy addition which allows the soup to be stirred by the appliance at regular intervals and can prevent sticking.

Cleaning:

Whilst using a soup maker certainly reduces the washing up, the unit itself does still need to be cleaned afterwards. Some appliances are easier to clean than others. Research how easily blades and elements of the unit can be removed for cleaning and again pay attention to reviews of those who have already purchased.

 Tips For Using Your Soup Maker

- Prepare all your ingredients first.
- Use hot stock in recipes, not cold.
- Cut your ingredients into small bite size pieces before adding to the soup maker.
- To prevent sticking use a little oil when sautéing.
- Do not use frozen ingredients as this will increase cooking times. Allow any frozen ingredients to thaw first.
- Do not use any meat with bones in the soup maker
- Do not use any seafood which are still in their shells in the soup maker
- If you have a jug/kettle style soup maker do not use raw meat or seafood – only cooked.
- If fitted, use the stir function regularly.
- Always make sure the lid is tightly closed and fastened before cooking.
- Follow the manufacturer's safety guidelines when using the appliance, particularly when opening the

lid after or during cooking, which may release scalding steam.

- Do not overfill your appliance. Pay careful attention to the capacity of your machine and the fill level markers. There are different levels for cold and hot liquids.

- Be careful of fully immersing your jug in water as this may result in short-circuiting the machine. Allow the soup maker to fully cool before attempting to clean. Heating plates and blades may still be very hot.

- Most soup makers are not dishwasher safe so must be cleaned manually. Warm soapy water should be sufficient. If the heating plate has become burned, soak in hot soapy water for longer and use a coarse sponge to remove. Avoid using any harsh cleaning products or scouring pads, as these will damage the surface of the heating plate.

- Read the manufactures instructions and guidelines for your appliance thoroughly before using. These will provide information, tips and safety guidelines specific to your product and should be adhered to in order to get the best out of your appliance.

All Recipes Are A Guide Only

All the recipes in this book are a guide only. You may need to alter quantities and cooking times to suit your own appliance – do not overfill your soup maker.

Consistency is also a question of personal preference. Some recipes suggest the best consistency to use. Feel free to experiment by adding more or less liquid to suit your own taste.

Skinny

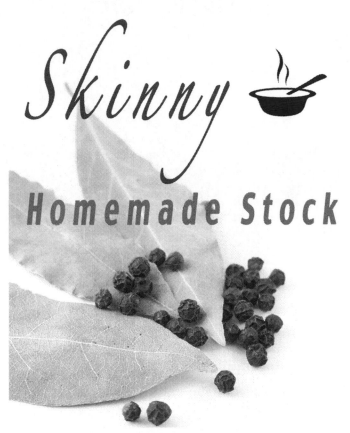

Homemade Stock

Homemade stock is not essential for any soup making, but if you fancy having a go you will find it can add additional depth of taste and further improve the flavour of some dishes. Having said that, shop bought stock has vastly improved in recent times and you may well decide making your own stock isn't worth the time for the comparable result. If you do use shop bought stock (which most people do) avoid buying budget options and anything too high in sodium.

Use a large pan rather than your soup maker as you will want to make bigger quantities.

Basic Vegetable Stock

Ingredients:

1 tbsp olive oil
1 onion, chopped
1 leek, chopped
1 carrot, chopped
1 small bulb fennel, chopped
3 garlic cloves, crushed
1 tbsp black peppercorns

75g/3oz mushrooms
2 sticks celery, chopped
3 tomatoes, diced
2 tbsp freshly chopped flat leaf parsley
2 bay leaves
3lt/12 cups water

Method:

Gently sauté the onions, leeks, carrots and fennel in the olive oil for a few minutes in a large lidded saucepan. Add all the other ingredients, cover and bring to the boil. Leave to gently simmer for 20 minutes with the lid on. Allow to cool for a little while. Pour the contents through a sieve and store the finished stock liquid in the fridge for a couple of days or freeze in batches.

Basic Chicken Stock

Ingredients:

1 tbsp olive oil
1 left over roast chicken carcass
2 carrots, chopped
2 onions, halved
2 stalks celery, chopped

10 black peppercorns
2 bay leaves
2 tbsp freshly chopped parsley
1 tsp freshly chopped thyme
3lt/12 cups water

Method:

Gently sauté the onions, carrots and celery in the olive oil for a few minutes in a large lidded saucepan. Break the chicken carcass up into pieces and add to the pan along with all the other ingredients, cover and bring to the boil. Leave to very gently simmer for 1hr with the lid on. Allow to cool for a little while. Pour the contents through a sieve and store the finished stock liquid in the fridge for a couple of days or freeze in batches. You may find you need to skim a little fat from the top of the stock after cooking.

Basic Fish Stock

Ingredients:

1 tbsp olive oil
450g/1lb fish bones, heads carcasses etc (avoid oily fish when making stock)
4 leeks, chopped

1 fennel bulb, chopped
4 carrots, chopped
2 tbsp freshly chopped parsley
250ml/1 cup dry white wine
2.5lt/10 cups water

Method:

Gently sauté the carrots, leeks and fennel in the olive oil for a few minutes in a large lidded saucepan. Clean the fish bones to ensure there is no blood as this can 'spoil' the stock. Add all the other ingredients, cover and bring to the boil. Leave to very gently simmer for 1hr with the lid on. Allow to cool for a little while. Pour the contents through a sieve and store the finished stock liquid in the fridge for a couple of days or freeze in batches. You may find you need to skim a little fat from the top of the stock after cooking.

Skinny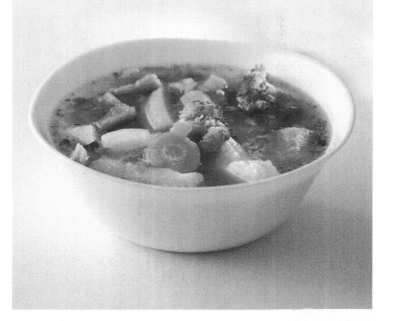

Vegetable &
Vegetarian Soups

Summer Salad Vegetable Soup
Serves 4

129 CALORIES PER SERVING

Ingredients:

1 tbsp olive oil
250g/9oz courgettes/zucchini, chopped
250g/9oz fresh peas
125g/4oz chard, chopped
1 small bunch spring onions/scallions, chopped
2 celery stalks, chopped

1 fennel bulb (aprox 250g), chopped
1 romaine lettuce, shredded
750ml/3 cups vegetable stock
2 tbsp freshly chopped garden herbs (parsley, basil & mint is a good combination)
Salt & pepper to taste

Method:

- Choose your preferred blend function, if required. Otherwise decide on your consistency at the end of cooking and then blend.
- If your soup maker has a browning function, add the olive oil and onions first and leave to brown for a few minutes.

Add all the ingredients, except the shredded lettuce, to the soup maker. Cover and leave to cook on high for 40 minutes. Ensure all the ingredients are well combined, tender and piping hot. Blend to your preferred consistency (or leave your machine to do this as programmed). Add the shredded lettuce, stir and leave to warm through for a further 2-3 minutes. Adjust the seasoning and serve.

This summery soup is perfect for showcasing the best of the vegetable garden. Feel free to substitute whichever summer vegetables you have to hand.

Mexican Lime, Bean & Tomato Soup
Serves 4

144
CALORIES
PER SERVING

Ingredients:

1 tbsp olive oil
2 garlic cloves, crushed
1 red chilli, deseeded and chopped
1 red onion, chopped
250ml/1 cup vegetable stock
250ml/1 cup tomato passata/sieved tomatoes
½ tsp each ground cumin, paprika & brown sugar

125g/4oz vine ripened tomatoes, chopped
200g/7oz black eyed beans
2 tbsp lime juice
3 tbsp freshly chopped coriander/cilantro
Salt & pepper to taste

Method:

- Choose your preferred blend function, if required. Otherwise decide on your consistency at the end of cooking and then blend.
- If your soup maker has a browning function, add the olive oil and onions first and leave to brown for a few minutes.

Add all the ingredients to the soup maker, except the lime juice. Cover and leave to cook on high for 30 minutes. Ensure all the ingredients are well combined, tender and piping hot. Blend to your preferred consistency (or leave your machine to do this as programmed). Stir through the lime juice, adjust the seasoning and serve.

Add some additional chilli to this this soup if you prefer more spice. This soup is best served as chunky as possible to keep the majority of the beans intact. Delicious served with a dollop of sour cream.

Pea, Parsley & Mint Soup
Serves 4

131 CALORIES PER SERVING

Ingredients:

1 tbsp olive oil
1 onion, chopped
1 tsp dried thyme
750ml/3 cups vegetable stock
400g/14oz peas fresh or frozen
(and thawed)

2 tbsp each freshly chopped
flat leaf parsley & mint
Salt & pepper to taste

Method:

- Choose your preferred blend function, if required. Otherwise decide on your consistency at the end of cooking and then blend.
- If your soup maker has a browning function, add the olive oil and onions first and leave to brown for a few minutes.

Add all the ingredients to the soup maker. Cover and leave to cook on high for 30 minutes. Ensure all the ingredients are well combined, tender and piping hot. Blend to your preferred consistency (or leave your machine to do this as programmed). Adjust the seasoning and serve.

It's possible to eat this soup chilled if you prefer. A swirl of olive oil or single cream just before serving also adds an extra dimension.

Celeriac & Orange Soup
Serves 4

103 CALORIES PER SERVING

Ingredients:

1 tbsp olive oil
1 onion, chopped
1 fennel bulb (aprox 500g), chopped
450g/1lb celeriac, chopped

750ml/3 cups vegetable stock
4 tbsp fat free Greek yoghurt
Zest of 1 large orange
Salt & pepper to taste

Method:

- Choose your preferred blend function, if required. Otherwise decide on your consistency at the end of cooking and then blend.
- If your soup maker has a browning function, add the olive oil and onions first and leave to brown for a few minutes.

Add all the ingredients to the soup maker, except the yoghurt. Cover and leave to cook on high for 30 minutes. Ensure all the ingredients are well combined, tender and piping hot. Blend to your preferred consistency (or leave your machine to do this as programmed). Adjust the seasoning and serve with a tbsp of yoghurt dolloped in the centre of each bowl of soup.

Celeriac & fennel form a great combination in soups. Their delicious and unusual taste is lightened here with the orange zest.

Mushroom, Cream & Herb Soup

Serves 4

150
CALORIES
PER SERVING

Ingredients:

1 tbsp olive oil
1 leek, chopped
750ml/3 cups vegetable stock
450g/1lb chestnut mushrooms, chopped
1 garlic clove, crushed

120ml/½ cup single cream
½ tsp dried thyme
¼ tsp ground nutmeg
1 tbsp plain/all-purpose flour
2 tbsp finely chopped chives, to serve

Method:

- Choose your preferred blend function, if required. Otherwise decide on your consistency at the end of cooking and then blend.
- If your soup maker has a browning function, add the olive oil and leeks first and leave to brown for a few minutes.

Add all the ingredients to the soup maker except the cream and chives. Cover and leave to cook on high for 30 minutes. Ensure all the ingredients are well combined, tender and piping hot. Blend to your preferred consistency (or leave your machine to do this as programmed). Stir through the cream, adjust the seasoning and serve with the chopped chives sprinkled on top.

It's fine to substitute whichever mushrooms you have to hand for this soup. You could also try some rehydrated chopped dried mushrooms to give a deeper flavour.

Fresh Ginger, Garlic & Parsnip Soup

Serves 4

142 CALORIES PER SERVING

Ingredients:

1 tbsp olive oil
1 onion, chopped
4 garlic cloves, crushed
1 tbsp freshly grated ginger
½ tsp each ground cumin &
paprika

500g/1lb 2oz parsnips, peeled
& chopped
500ml/2 cups vegetable stock
250ml/1 cup semi-skimmed
milk
Salt & pepper to taste

Method:

- Choose your preferred blend function, if required. Otherwise decide on your consistency at the end of cooking and then blend.
- If your soup maker has a browning function, add the olive oil and onions first and leave to brown for a few minutes.

Add all the ingredients to the soup maker. Cover and leave to cook on high for 30 minutes. Ensure all the ingredients are well combined, tender and piping hot. Blend to your preferred consistency (or leave your machine to do this as programmed). Adjust the seasoning and serve.

Parsnips have a natural sweetness to them which is beautifully complemented by the earthy fieriness of the fresh ginger.

Sweet Potato & Coconut Milk Soup
Serves 4

235
CALORIES
PER SERVING

Ingredients:

1 tbsp olive oil
2 onions, chopped
3 garlic cloves, crushed
1 tbsp freshly grated ginger
½ tsp crushed chilli flakes
(more or less to taste)
1 tbsp medium curry powder
500g/1lb 2oz sweet potatoes,
peeled & cubed

500ml/2 cups vegetable stock
250ml/1 cup coconut milk
1 tbsp lime juice
1 tbsp freshly chopped
coriander/cilantro
Salt & pepper to taste

Method:

- Choose your preferred blend function, if required. Otherwise decide on your consistency at the end of cooking and then blend.
- If your soup maker has a browning function, add the olive oil and onions first and leave to brown for a few minutes.

Add all the ingredients, except the coconut milk to the soup maker. Cover and leave to cook on high for 30 minutes. Ensure all the ingredients are well combined, tender and piping hot. Blend to your preferred consistency (or leave your machine to do this as programmed). Stir through the coconut milk and leave to gently warm through. Adjust the seasoning and serve.

Coconut milk works really well in soup. If you prefer an even more silky and rich texture use coconut cream instead of coconut milk.

28

Chickpea, Coriander & Cumin Seed Soup

Serves 4

142 CALORIES PER SERVING

Ingredients:

1 tbsp olive oil
300g/11oz tinned chickpeas, drained
1 red chilli, deseeded and chopped
2 tsp coriander/cilantro seeds, crushed with a pestle & mortar
2 tsp cumin seeds, crushed with a pestle & mortar

4 cloves garlic, crushed
1 tsp ground turmeric
750ml/3cups vegetable stock
Zest of 1 lemon
2 tbsp lemon juice
Salt & pepper to taste

Method:

- Choose your preferred blend function, if required. Otherwise decide on your consistency at the end of cooking and then blend.

Add all the ingredients to the soup maker, except the lemon juice. Cover and leave to cook on high for 30 minutes. Ensure all the ingredients are well combined, tender and piping hot. Blend to your preferred consistency (or leave your machine to do this as programmed). Add the lemon juice, adjust the seasoning and serve.

The spices in this delicious recipe have a real Mexican feel to them. Stirring through the lemon juice just before serving adds a great 'spark' to this warming soup.

29

Artichoke & Carrot Soup
Serves 4

120 CALORIES PER SERVING

Ingredients:

1 tbsp olive oil
300g/11oz carrots, chopped
300g/11oz Jerusalem artichokes
1 celery stalk, chopped

1 onion, chopped
750ml/3 cups vegetable stock
Pinch saffron threads
Salt & pepper to taste

Method:

- Choose your preferred blend function, if required. Otherwise decide on your consistency at the end of cooking and then blend.
- If your soup maker has a browning function, add the olive oil and onions first and leave to brown for a few minutes.

Add all the ingredients to the soup maker. Cover and leave to cook on high for 30 minutes. Ensure all the ingredients are well combined, tender and piping hot. Blend to your preferred consistency (or leave your machine to do this as programmed). Adjust the seasoning and serve.

Artichokes are an often overlooked vegetable. They look slightly daunting but are very simple to cook with and provide a distinctive taste which is complemented by the saffron threads.

Creamy Celery Soup
Serves 4

170 CALORIES PER SERVING

Ingredients:

1 tbsp olive oil
350g/12oz celery stalks, chopped
125g/4oz potatoes, peeled and cubed
1 leek, chopped

250ml/1 cup vegetable stock
½ tsp celery seeds
250ml/1 cup whole milk
250ml/1 cup single cream
Salt & pepper to taste

Method:

- Choose your preferred blend function, if required. Otherwise decide on your consistency at the end of cooking and then blend.
- If your soup maker has a browning function, add the olive oil and leeks first and leave to brown for a few minutes.

Add all the ingredients to the soup maker, except the cream. Cover and leave to cook on high for 30 minutes. Ensure all the ingredients are well combined, tender and piping hot. Blend to your preferred consistency (or leave your machine to do this as programmed). Stir through the cream and leave to warm for minute or two. Adjust the seasoning and serve.

Celery seeds are actually very small fruit, which add a lovely depth of taste to this delicate soup. When preparing this recipe you could reserve the celery leaves, chop and use as a garnish when serving.

Watercress & Leek Soup
Serves 4

147
CALORIES
PER SERVING

Ingredients:

1 tbsp olive oil
125g/4oz watercress, chopped
3 leeks, chopped
350g/12oz potatoes, peeled &
cut into very small cubes

750ml/3 cups vegetable stock
4 tbsp crème fraiche
Salt & pepper to taste

Method:

- Choose your preferred blend function, if required. Otherwise decide on your consistency at the end of cooking and then blend.
- If your soup maker has a browning function, add the olive oil and leeks first and leave to brown for a few minutes.

Add all the ingredients to the soup maker, except the crème fraiche. Cover and leave to cook on high for 20 minutes. Ensure all the ingredients are well combined, tender and piping hot. Blend to your preferred consistency (or leave your machine to do this as programmed). Adjust the seasoning and serve with a tbsp of crème fraiche dolloped in the centre of each bowl of soup.

Watercress is believed to have many health benefits. Used as a traditional remedy to allergies it is also thought to aid weight loss!

Cauliflower & Roquefort Cheese Soup

220 CALORIES PER SERVING

Serves 4

Ingredients:

1 tbsp olive oil
1 onion, chopped
750ml/3 cups vegetable stock
1 stick celery, chopped
1 leek, chopped
125g/4oz potatoes, peeled & cubed
1 bay leaf (remove before blending)

450g/1lb cauliflower florets
120ml/½ cup single cream
50g/2oz Roquefort cheese (or vegetarian alternative)
2 tbsp freshly chopped chives
Salt & pepper to taste

Method:

- Choose your preferred blend function, if required. Otherwise decide on your consistency at the end of cooking and then blend.
- If your soup maker has a browning function, add the olive oil, leek and onions first and leave to brown for a few minutes.

Add all the ingredients to the soup maker except the cream and chives. Cover and leave to cook on high for 30 minutes. Ensure all the ingredients are well combined, tender and piping hot. Remove the bay leaf and blend to your preferred consistency (or leave your machine to do this as programmed). Stir through the cream and leave to warm through for a minute or two. Adjust the seasoning and serve with the chopped chives sprinkled on top.

The Roquefort cheese in this recipe can be substituted for stilton or extra mature cheddar if you prefer.

Caramelised French Onion Soup

Serves 4

160 CALORIES PER SERVING

Ingredients:

1 tbsp olive oil
500g/1lb 2oz onions, sliced
3 cloves garlic, crushed
1 tsp brown sugar

250ml/1 cup dry white wine
500ml/2 cups vegetable stock
Salt & pepper to taste

Method:

- Choose your preferred blend function, if required. Otherwise decide on your consistency at the end of cooking and then blend.
- If your soup maker has a browning function, add the olive oil and onions and sugar first and leave to brown for a few minutes.

Add all the ingredients to the soup maker. Cover and leave to cook on high for 30 minutes. Ensure all the ingredients are well combined, tender and piping hot. Blend to your preferred consistency (or leave your machine to do this as programmed). Adjust the seasoning and serve.

This mellow sweet soup is a French classic - delicious served with crusty bread and/or cheese croutons.

Tuscan Ditalini Soup
Serves 4

180
CALORIES
PER SERVING

Ingredients:

1 tbsp olive oil
225g/8oz tinned Italian beans
eg. borlotti or cannellini
125g/4oz ditalini pasta
1 tsp dried rosemary

3 garlic cloves, crushed
2 tbsp tomato puree/paste
1 onion, chopped
750ml/3 cups vegetable stock
Salt & pepper to taste

Method:

- Choose your preferred blend function, if required. Otherwise decide on your consistency at the end of cooking and then blend.
- If your soup maker has a browning function, add the olive oil and onions first and leave to brown for a few minutes.

Add all the ingredients to the soup maker. Cover and leave to cook on high for 30 minutes. Ensure all the ingredients are well combined, tender and piping hot. Blend to your preferred consistency (or leave your machine to do this as programmed). Adjust the seasoning and serve.

Ditalini is a short macaroni style pasta. This soup is best left as chunky as possible to keep the pasta shapes intact. Feel free to substitute with any other similar small pasta and serve with lots of freshly grated parmesan cheese (or vegetarian alternative).

Honeyed Carrot Soup
Serves 4

Ingredients:

1 tbsp olive oil
2 leeks, sliced
650g/1lb 7oz carrots, chopped
2 tsp clear runny honey

1 bay leaf (remove before blending)
750ml/3 cups vegetable stock
Salt & pepper to taste

Method:

- Choose your preferred blend function, if required. Otherwise decide on your consistency at the end of cooking and then blend.
- If your soup maker has a browning function, add the olive oil and leeks first and leave to brown for a few minutes.

Add all the ingredients to the soup maker. Cover and leave to cook on high for 30 minutes. Ensure all the ingredients are well combined, tender and piping hot. Remove the bay leaf and blend to your preferred consistency (or leave your machine to do this as programmed). Adjust the seasoning and serve.

This honey-sweet soup is always a success with the whole family. Add a pinch of crushed chilli flakes when serving for a little kick, plus a swirl of single cream is lovely too.

Tasty Triple Onion & Mustard Soup
Serves 4

211 CALORIES PER SERVING

Ingredients:

2 tbsp olive oil
1 tbsp djion mustard
200g/7oz red onions
200g/7oz shallots
300g/11oz regular white onions

3 tsp plain/all purpose flour
2 tsp dried thyme
750ml/3 cups cups vegetable stock
Salt & pepper to taste

Method:

- Choose your preferred blend function, if required. Otherwise decide on your consistency at the end of cooking and then blend.
- If your soup maker has a browning function, add the olive oil and onions first and leave to brown for a few minutes.

Add all the ingredients to the soup maker. Cover and leave to cook on high for 30 minutes. Ensure all the ingredients are well combined, tender and piping hot. Blend to your preferred consistency (or leave your machine to do this as programmed). Adjust the seasoning and serve.

It's fine to alter the balance of onions in this dish. You could also add some spring onions/scallions as a garnish and also consider increasing the mustard to suit your taste.

Sweet Squash & Sunflower Seed Soup

Serves 4

260 CALORIES PER SERVING

Ingredients:

1 tbsp olive oil
1 tbsp sunflower seeds, chopped
450g/1lb butternut squash flesh, peeled and cubed

200g/7oz potatoes, peeled and cubed
750ml/3 cups vegetable stock
60ml/ ½ cup single cream
Salt & pepper to taste

Method:

- Choose your preferred blend function, if required. Otherwise decide on your consistency at the end of cooking and then blend.

Add all the ingredients to the soup maker, except the sunflower seeds and cream. Cover and leave to cook on high for 40 minutes. Ensure all the ingredients are well combined, tender and piping hot. Blend to your preferred consistency (or leave your machine to do this as programmed). Stir through the cream and leave to warm for a minute or two. Adjust the seasoning and serve with the sunflower seeds sprinkled on top.

The sunflower seeds in this recipe are best toasted for the garnish but you can serve them raw too if you like.

Best Ever Vegetable Dhal Soup

Serves 4

230 CALORIES PER SERVING

Ingredients:

1 tbsp olive oil
3 garlic cloves, crushed
1 onion, chopped
1 tsp each ground turmeric, cumin, coriander/cilantro
½ tsp each cayenne pepper, ground ginger & garam masala
200g/7oz red lentils

200g/7oz cauliflower florets
125g/4oz sweet potato, peeled & cubed
125g/4oz spinach leaves, chopped
750ml/3 cups vegetable stock
1 tbsp lemon juice
Salt & pepper to taste

Method:

- Choose your preferred blend function, if required. Otherwise decide on your consistency at the end of cooking and then blend.
- If your soup maker has a browning function, add the olive oil and onions first and leave to brown for a few minutes.

Add all the ingredients to the soup maker, except the lemon juice. Cover and leave to cook on high for 40 minutes. Ensure all the ingredients are well combined, tender and piping hot. Blend to your preferred consistency (or leave your machine to do this as programmed). Stir through the lemon juice, adjust the seasoning and serve.

Dahl is one of the world's most popular dishes and is eaten by some families at almost every mealtime. This 'soupy' version can be spiced up with additional cayenne pepper or hot chilli powder and garnished with fresh chopped coriander/cilantro as preferred.

Pak Choi & Spicy Spring-Green Soup
Serves 4

130 CALORIES PER SERVING

Ingredients:

750ml/3 cups vegetable stock
250g/9oz pak choi, sliced
75g/3oz purple sprouting broccoli, finely chopped
75g/3oz potatoes, peeled & cut into very small cubes
75g/3 oz fresh peas
1 onion, chopped

2 tsp brown sugar
1 leek, chopped
2 tsp freshly grated ginger
1 red chilli, deseeded and chopped
2 garlic cloves, crushed
Salt & pepper to taste

Method:

- Choose your preferred blend function, if required. Otherwise decide on your consistency at the end of cooking and then blend.

Add all the ingredients to the soup maker, except for a handful of the pak choi. Cover and leave to cook on high for 20 minutes. Ensure all the ingredients are well combined, tender and piping hot. Blend to your preferred consistency (or leave your machine to do this as programmed). Add the reserved pak choi and cook for a further 2-3 minutes. Adjust the seasoning and serve.

Pak choi is a fantastic Asian vegetable which is versatile and surprisingly easy to grow even in some of the toughest climates.

Seasoned White Bean Soup
Serves 4

240
CALORIES
PER SERVING

Ingredients:

1 tbsp olive oil
250g/9oz dried cannellini beans, pre soaked
1 onion, chopped
1 celery stalk, chopped
3 garlic cloves, crushed
2 ripe tomatoes, chopped

1 bay leaf (removed before blending)
1 tbsp dried thyme
1 tbsp freshly chopped parsley
750ml/3 cups vegetable stock
Salt & pepper to taste

Method:

- Choose your preferred blend function, if required. Otherwise decide on your consistency at the end of cooking and then blend.
- If your soup maker has a browning function, add the olive oil and onions first and leave to brown for a few minutes.

Add all the ingredients to the soup maker, except the chopped parsley. Cover and leave to cook on high for 20 minutes. Ensure all the ingredients are well combined, tender and piping hot. Remove the bay leaf. Blend to your preferred consistency (or leave your machine to do this as programmed). Adjust the seasoning and serve with the chopped parsley sprinkled over the top.

Tinned cannellini, or any other white bean, will work just as well with this recipe if you don't have time to pre-soak. Season this soup really well with lots of freshly ground black pepper to get the balance right.

Tarka-Dhal Soup
Serves 4

2 4 0
CALORIES
PER SERVING

Ingredients:

1 tbsp olive oil
75g/3oz yellow split peas
125g/4oz red lentils
750ml/3 cups vegetable stock
4 garlic cloves, crushed
2 fresh tomatoes, chopped
1 tsp ground turmeric
2 red or green chillies,
deseeded and finely chopped

2 onions, chopped
½ tsp each mustard seeds &
onions seeds
½ tsp crushed chilli flakes
1 tbsp each freshly chopped
coriander/cilantro & mint
Salt & pepper to taste

Method:

- Choose your preferred blend function, if required. Otherwise decide on your consistency at the end of cooking and then blend.
- If your soup maker has a browning function, add the olive oil and onions first and leave to brown for a few minutes.

Add all the ingredients to the soup maker, except the chopped mint and coriander. Cover and leave to cook on high for 30 minutes. Ensure all the ingredients are well combined, tender and piping hot. Blend to your preferred consistency (or leave your machine to do this as programmed). Adjust the seasoning and serve with the chopped mint & coriander sprinkled over the top.

To make this a more authentic Indian soup dish heat 3 tbsp olive oil in a sauce pan with 2 tsp mustard seeds until they pop. Pour this hot oil onto each soup bowl before serving and stir.

Pea & Pumpkin Soup
Serves 4

230 CALORIES PER SERVING

Ingredients:

1 tbsp olive oil
750ml/3 cups vegetable stock
225g/8oz pumpkin flesh, chopped
225g/8oz dried split peas, pre soaked

1 onion, chopped
1 stalk celery, chopped
1 tsp dried rosemary
2 tsp ground cumin
½ tsp crushed chilli flakes
Salt & pepper to taste

Method:

- Choose your preferred blend function, if required. Otherwise decide on your consistency at the end of cooking and then blend.
- If your soup maker has a browning function, add the olive oil and onions first and leave to brown for a few minutes.

Add all the ingredients to the soup maker. Cover and leave to cook on high for 30 minutes. Ensure all the ingredients are well combined, tender and piping hot. Blend to your preferred consistency (or leave your machine to do this as programmed). Adjust the seasoning and serve.

This soup is equally good using butternut squash and it's also nice with a little single cream swirled through before serving.

Yam Soup
Serves 4

Ingredients:

1 tbsp olive oil
175g/6oz yam, peeled & cubed
750ml/3 cups vegetable stock
1 onion, chopped
1 celery stick, chopped
2 carrots, chopped
2 garlic cloves, crushed

2 un-ripened green bananas, sliced
1 tsp each dried thyme & oregano
50g/2oz red lentils
Salt & pepper to taste

Method:

• Choose your preferred blend function, if required. Otherwise decide on your consistency at the end of cooking and then blend.
• If your soup maker has a browning function, add the olive oil and onions first and leave to brown for a few minutes

Add all the ingredients to the soup maker. Cover and leave to cook on high for 30 minutes. Ensure all the ingredients are well combined, tender and piping hot. Blend to your preferred consistency (or leave your machine to do this as programmed). Adjust the seasoning and serve.

Sweet potato will work fine in this recipe if yams are not easily available. Leave the soup as chunky as you can to enjoy it at its best.

Ciabatta Soup
Serves 4

295 CALORIES PER SERVING

Ingredients:

1 tbsp olive oil
1 onion, chopped
450g/1lb vine ripened tomatoes
750ml/3 cups vegetable stock
4 garlic cloves, crushed

1 tsp brown sugar
125g/4oz ciabatta bread, cubed
Large bunch fresh basil, chopped
Salt & pepper to taste

Method:

- Choose your preferred blend function, if required. Otherwise decide on your consistency at the end of cooking and then blend.
- If your soup maker has a browning function, add the olive oil and onions first and leave to brown for a few minutes.

Add all the ingredients to the soup maker, reserve a little chopped basil for garnish. Cover and leave to cook on high for 30 minutes. Ensure all the ingredients are well combined, tender and piping hot. Blend to your preferred consistency (or leave your machine to do this as programmed). Adjust the seasoning and serve with chopped basil sprinkled over the top.

Any firm crusty bread can be substituted in this recipe. Use bread which is as stale as possible to make it nice and hard.

Cheesy Leek Soup
Serves 4

190 CALORIES PER SERVING

Ingredients:

1 tbsp olive oil
3 leeks, chopped
750ml/3 cups vegetable stock
1 tbsp Dijon mustard
75g/3oz creamy blue cheese
(or vegetarian alternative)

3 tbsp freshly chopped chives
1 tbsp cornflour mixed with
a little warm water to form a
paste

Method:

- Choose your preferred blend function, if required. Otherwise decide on your consistency at the end of cooking and then blend.
- If your soup maker has a browning function, add the olive oil and leeks first and leave to brown for a few minutes.

Add all the ingredients to the soup maker, except the chopped chives. Cover and leave to cook on high for 20 minutes. Ensure all the ingredients are well combined, tender and piping hot. Blend to your preferred consistency (or leave your machine to do this as programmed). Adjust the seasoning and serve with chopped chives sprinkled over the top.

Use whichever blue cheese you prefer in this recipe. Feel free to add a little extra cheese crumbled over the top of each soup bowl as a garnish.

Creamy Parsnip & Cumin Soup
Serves 4

280 CALORIES PER SERVING

Ingredients:

1 tbsp olive oil
450g/1lb parsnips, chopped
2 onions, chopped
3 garlic cloves, crushed
2 tsp ground cumin

1 tsp ground coriander/cilantro
750ml/3 cups vegetable stock
120ml/ ½ cup single cream
3 tbsp freshly chopped chives
Salt & pepper to taste

Method:

• Choose your preferred blend function, if required. Otherwise decide on your consistency at the end of cooking and then blend.

• If your soup maker has a browning function, add the olive oil and onions first and leave to brown for a few minutes.

Add all the ingredients to the soup maker, except the chopped chives and cream. Cover and leave to cook on high for 30 minutes. Ensure all the ingredients are well combined, tender and piping hot. Blend to your preferred consistency (or leave your machine to do this as programmed). Stir through the cream and leave to warm for a minute or two. Adjust the seasoning and serve with chopped chives sprinkled over the top.

A dollop of sour cream along with some freshly chopped coriander/cilantro also adds a lovely garnish to this creamy soup.

Macadamia Nut & French Bean Soup
Serves 4

Ingredients:

225g/8oz French beans, chopped
2 garlic cloves, crushed
200g/7oz potatoes, peeled & finely chopped
1 tsp anchovy paste
2 onions, chopped
1 bay leaf (removed before blending)

250ml/1 cup coconut milk
500ml/2 cups vegetable stock
2 tbsp macadamia nuts, chopped
200g/7oz beansprouts
Salt & pepper to taste

Method:

• Choose your preferred blend function, if required. Otherwise decide on your consistency at the end of cooking and then blend.

Add all the ingredients to the soup maker, except the coconut milk, nuts and beansprouts. Cover and leave to cook on high for 20 minutes. Ensure all the ingredients are well combined tender and piping hot. Blend to your preferred consistency (or leave your machine to do this as programmed). Stir through the coconut milk and beansprouts and leave to warm through for a few minutes. Adjust the seasoning and serve with the nuts sprinkled on top.

You could choose to add the beansprouts at the end of cooking and serve as a raw crunchy garnish on top of the soup.

Potato & Parsley Soup
Serves 4

180 CALORIES PER SERVING

Ingredients:

1 tbsp olive oil
50g/2oz long grain rice
750ml/3 cups vegetable stock
1 large bunch flat leaf parsley, finely chopped

1 onion, chopped
1 leek, chopped
125g/4oz potatoes, peeled & cubed
Salt & pepper to taste

Method:

- Choose your preferred blend function, if required. Otherwise decide on your consistency at the end of cooking and then blend.
- If your soup maker has a browning function, add the olive oil, onions and leeks first and leave to brown for a few minutes.

Add all the ingredients to the soup maker. Cover and leave to cook on high for 20 minutes. Ensure all the ingredients are well combined, tender and piping hot. Blend to your preferred consistency (or leave your machine to do this as programmed). Adjust the seasoning and serve.

You could try making this soup with another member of the parsley family – chervil which will give you a slightly different taste.

Gouda & Celeriac Soup
Serves 4

290
CALORIES
PER SERVING

Ingredients:

1 tbsp olive oil
1 onion, chopped
200g/7oz celeriac, peeled & finely chopped
75g/3oz grated gouda cheese (or vegetarian alternative)
500ml/2 cups vegetable stock

250ml/1 cup semi skimmed milk
1 tbsp cornflour mixed with a little warm water to form a paste
Salt & pepper to taste

Method:

- Choose your preferred blend function, if required. Otherwise decide on your consistency at the end of cooking and then blend.
- If your soup maker has a browning function, add the olive oil and onions first and leave to brown for a few minutes.

Add all the ingredients to the soup maker. Cover and leave to cook on low for 30-40 minutes. Ensure all the ingredients are well combined, tender and piping hot. Blend to your preferred consistency (or leave your machine to do this as programmed). Adjust the seasoning and serve.

Turnips make a suitable alternative to celeriac if needed. Also a little single cream swirled over the top before serving is lovely.

Skinny
Meat &
Poultry Soups

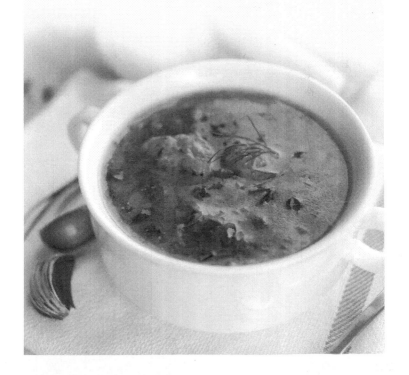

Chicken & Asparagus Soup

Serves 4

230
CALORIES
PER SERVING

Ingredients:

1 tbsp olive oil
125g/4oz fresh asparagus, trimmed and roughly chopped
750ml/3 cups chicken stock
250ml/1 cup dry white wine
2 garlic cloves, crushed
1 tsp each freshly chopped flat leaf parsley & dill

350g/12oz skinless chicken breast, chopped
50g/2oz rice noodles
1 leek, chopped
1 onion, chopped
Salt & pepper to taste

Method:

- Choose your preferred blend function, if required. Otherwise decide on your consistency at the end of cooking and then blend.
- Use cooked chicken in this recipe unless your soup maker is suitable for raw meat and has a browning function. If it does so add the olive oil, onions, leeks & chicken first. Leave to cook for 15 minutes or until the chicken is cooked through and then follow the method below.

Add all the ingredients to the soup maker. Cover and leave to cook on high for 30 minutes. Ensure all the ingredients are well combined, tender and piping hot. Blend to your preferred consistency (or leave your machine to do this as programmed). Adjust the seasoning and serve.

Use the freshest asparagus you can find for this recipe to make use of its natural seasonal sweetness.

Original Chicken & Leek Soup

Serves 4

Ingredients:

1 tbsp olive oil
275g/10oz skinless chicken breast, cut into chunks
1 tsp each dried thyme, rosemary & basil

2 leeks, chopped
1lt/4 cups chicken stock
10 dried prunes, chopped
Salt & pepper to taste

Method:

- Choose your preferred blend function, if required. Otherwise decide on your consistency at the end of cooking and then blend.
- Use cooked chicken in this recipe unless your soup maker is suitable for raw meat and has a browning function. If it does so add the olive oil, leeks & chicken first. Leave to cook for 15 minutes or until the chicken is cooked through and then follow the method below.

Add all the ingredients to the soup maker. Cover and leave to cook on high for 30 minutes. Ensure all the ingredients are well combined, tender and piping hot. Blend to your preferred consistency (or leave your machine to do this as programmed). Adjust the seasoning and serve.

You can use any number of herb combinations for this recipe. Put together a bouquet garni sachet if you like instead of the dried herbs suggested in the recipe. .

53

Beef and Pearl Barley Soup

Serves 4

Ingredients:

1 tbsp olive oil
225g/8oz lean sirloin beef, chopped
2 tsp dried mixed herbs
50g/2oz pre-soaked pearl barley

1 carrot, chopped
1 onion, chopped
1 leek, chopped
2 celery stalks, chopped
1lt/4 cups beef stock
Salt & pepper to taste

Method:

- Choose your preferred blend function, if required. Otherwise decide on your consistency at the end of cooking and then blend.
- Use cooked beef in this recipe unless your soup maker is suitable for raw meat and has a browning function. If it does so add the olive oil, leeks, onion & beef first. Leave to cook for 15 minutes or until the beef is cooked through and then follow the method below.

Add all the ingredients to the soup maker. Cover and leave to cook on high for 30 minutes. Ensure all the ingredients are well combined, tender and piping hot. Blend to your preferred consistency (or leave your machine to do this as programmed). Adjust the seasoning and serve.

The pearl barley thickens the soup and gives it a creamy texture. You can substitute spelt barley in place of pearl barley.

54

Chicken & Sweetcorn Soup
Serves 4

Ingredients:

1 tbsp olive oil
225g/8oz skinless chicken breast, chopped
200g/7oz sweetcorn (thaw if using frozen)
750ml/3 cups chicken stock
1 red (bell) pepper, finely chopped

1 tsp freshly chopped coriander/cilantro
1 onion, chopped
3 fresh tomatoes, chopped
2 tbsp tomato, puree/paste
Salt & pepper to taste

Method:

- Choose your preferred blend function, if required. Otherwise decide on your consistency at the end of cooking and then blend.
- Use cooked chicken in this recipe unless your soup maker is suitable for raw meat and has a browning function. If it does so add the olive oil, onions & chicken first. Leave to cook for 15 minutes or until the chicken is cooked through and then follow the method below.

Add all the ingredients to the soup maker. Cover and leave to cook on high for 30 minutes. Ensure all the ingredients are well combined, tender and piping hot. Blend to your preferred consistency (or leave your machine to do this as programmed). Adjust the seasoning and serve.

You could add oregano to this recipe and also substitute the fresh tomatoes for tinned chopped tomatoes if you wish.

Thai Chicken & Coconut Soup

Serves 4

240 CALORIES PER SERVING

Ingredients:

1 tsp olive oil
200g/7oz skinless chicken breast
250ml/1 cup reduced fat coconut milk
500ml/2 cups chicken stock
2 stalks fresh lemon grass, peeled & finely chopped
1 bunch spring onion/scallions, chopped

2 tbsp lime juice
1 tsp freshly grated ginger
1 tbsp soy sauce
1 tsp ground ginger
1 red chilli, deseeded and finely chopped
1 tbsp corn flour dissolved into a little warm water to form a paste
Salt & pepper to taste

Method:

- Choose your preferred blend function, if required. Otherwise decide on your consistency at the end of cooking and then blend.
- Use cooked chicken in this recipe unless your soup maker is suitable for raw meat and has a browning function. If it does so add the olive oil & chicken first. Leave to cook for 15 minutes or until the chicken is cooked through and then follow the method below.

Add all the ingredients to the soup maker, except the coconut milk and lime juice. Cover and leave to cook on high for 30 minutes. Ensure all the ingredients are well combined, tender and piping hot. Blend to your preferred consistency (or leave your machine to do this as programmed). Add the coconut milk, stir and leave to warm through for 2-3 minutes. Adjust the seasoning, add the lime juice and serve.

This simple Thai-inspired soup is a great combination of citrus flavours and robust spices.

Beef & Rice Soup
Serves 4

265
CALORIES
PER SERVING

Ingredients:

1 tbsp olive oil
1lt/4 cups beef stock
1 cinnamon stick, bashed
(remove before blending)
1 onion, chopped
200g/7oz lean sirloin beef,
chopped
1 star anise (remove before
blending)

2 tbsp soy sauce
2 tbsp tomato puree/paste
125g/4oz ready to use bamboo
shoots
125g/4oz long grain rice
60ml/ ¼ cup fresh orange juice
Salt & pepper to taste

Method:

- Choose your preferred blend function, if required. Otherwise decide on your consistency at the end of cooking and then blend.
- Use cooked beef in this recipe unless your soup maker is suitable for raw meat and has a browning function. If it does so add the olive oil, onions & beef first. Leave to cook for 15 minutes or until the beef is cooked through and then follow the method below.

Add all the ingredients to the soup maker, except the orange juice. Cover and leave to cook on high for 30 minutes. Ensure all the ingredients are well combined, tender and piping hot. Remove the cinnamon and star anise. Blend to your preferred consistency (or leave your machine to do this as programmed). Adjust the seasoning and serve.

Remember to remove the star anise and cinnamon stick before any blending as these will ruin the soup if left in.

Chicken & Anellini Pasta Soup
Serves 4

280 CALORIES PER SERVING

Ingredients:

1 tbsp olive oil
200g/7oz skinless chicken breast, chopped
1 onion, chopped
125g/4oz anellini pasta
2 carrots, chopped

125g/4oz cauliflower, cut into florets
750ml/3 cups chicken stock
2 tsp dried herbs
Salt & pepper to taste

Method:

Add the shredded cabbage and water to a pan and cook gently for 5 minutes or until the cabbage is cooked to your liking. Add the sugar, vinegar and salt and cook for a minute or two longer and serve. You may need to alter the balance of sugar, vinegar and salt to get the balance of sweet, sour and salty just right.

Anellini are very small pasta shapes which are great for soups, you can easily substitute for any other soup pasta.

The Original Chicken Broth
Serves 4

Ingredients:

1 tbsp olive oil
225g/8oz skinless chicken breast
50g/2oz pre-soaked dried peas
750ml/3 cups chicken broth
1 carrot, chopped

1 onion, chopped
1 leek, chopped
50g/2oz pearl barley
1 tsp freshly chopped thyme
2 stalks celery, chopped
Salt & pepper to taste

Method:

- Choose your preferred blend function, if required. Otherwise decide on your consistency at the end of cooking and then blend.
- Use cooked chicken in this recipe unless your soup maker is suitable for raw meat and has a browning function. If it does so add the olive oil, onions, leeks & chicken first. Leave to cook for 15 minutes or until the chicken is cooked through and then follow the method below.

Add all the ingredients to the soup maker. Cover and leave to cook on high for 30 minutes. Ensure all the ingredients are well combined, tender and piping hot. Blend to your preferred consistency (or leave your machine to do this as programmed). Adjust the seasoning and serve.

This is another soup which is best served chunky…. along with a large chunk of freshly baked crusty bread.

Ham & Pea Soup
Serves 4

298 CALORIES PER SERVING

Ingredients:

1 tbsp olive oil
750ml/3 cups chicken stock
225g/8oz dried split peas
1 onion, chopped
2 carrots, chopped
1 celery stalk, chopped

1 smoked cooked ham hock, meat stripped
1 tsp each dried oregano & thyme
½ tsp ground ginger
Salt & pepper to taste

Method:

- Choose your preferred blend function, if required. Otherwise decide on your consistency at the end of cooking and then blend.
- If your soup maker has a browning function, add the olive oil & onions first. Leave to cook for a few minutes and then follow the method below.

Add all the ingredients to the soup maker. Cover and leave to cook on low for 30 minutes. Ensure all the ingredients are well combined, tender and piping hot. Blend to your preferred consistency (or leave your machine to do this as programmed). Adjust the seasoning and serve.

A smoked ham hock is best but meat from an un-smoked hock would be fine too.

Pork Hot & Sour Soup

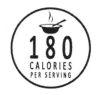

Serves 4

Ingredients:

1 tbsp olive oil
1 handful shitake mushrooms pre-soaked & chopped
200g/7oz pork tenderloin, chopped
75g/3oz ready to use bamboo shoots
125g/4oz tofu, cubed

1 tbsp tamarind paste
750ml/3 cups chicken stock
3 tbsp rice wine vinegar
1 tbsp soy sauce
½ tsp crushed chilli flakes
Bunch spring onions/scallions, chopped
Salt & pepper to taste

Method:

- Choose your preferred blend function, if required. Otherwise decide on your consistency at the end of cooking and then blend.
- Use cooked pork in this recipe unless your soup maker is suitable for raw meat and has a browning function. If it does so add the olive oil & pork first. Leave to cook for 15 minutes or until the pork is cooked through and then follow the method below.

Add all the ingredients to the soup maker. Cover and leave to cook on high for 30 minutes. Ensure all the ingredients are well combined, tender and piping hot. Blend to your preferred consistency (or leave your machine to do this as programmed). Adjust the seasoning and serve.

Feel free to add more crushed chilli flakes to this recipe if you prefer more 'heat'.

Lentil & Bacon Soup
Serves 4

230 CALORIES PER SERVING

Ingredients:

1 tbsp olive oil
1 onion, chopped
2 garlic cloves, crushed
150g/5oz lean back bacon, chopped
200g/7oz red lentils
750ml/3 cups chicken stock
3 fresh tomatoes, chopped

2 bay leaves (remove before blending)
¼ tsp ground all spice
125g/4oz potatoes, peeled & cubed
Bunch spring onions/scallions, chopped
Salt & pepper to taste

Method:

- Choose your preferred blend function, if required. Otherwise decide on your consistency at the end of cooking and then blend.
- Use cooked bacon in this recipe unless your soup maker is suitable for raw meat and has a browning function. If it does so add the olive oil, onions & bacon first. Leave to cook for 5-10 minutes or until the bacon is cooked through and then follow the method below.

Add all the ingredients to the soup maker. Cover and leave to cook on high for 50-60 minutes. Ensure all the ingredients are well combined, tender and piping hot. Remove the bay leaves. Blend to your preferred consistency (or leave your machine to do this as programmed). Adjust the seasoning and serve.

Serve with lots of freshly chopped flat leaf parsley and a swirl of single cream if you prefer a more luxurious texture.

Sherry Beef Soup
Serves 4

190 CALORIES PER SERVING

Ingredients:

1 tbsp olive oil
60ml/ ¼ cup dry sherry
250g/9oz frying steak, finely chopped
125g/4oz potatoes, peeled & cubed
1 leek, chopped

1 onion, chopped
1 carrot, chopped
1 celery stalk, chopped
750ml/3 cups beef stock
2 tsp dried mixed herbs
Salt & pepper to taste

Method:

- Choose your preferred blend function, if required. Otherwise decide on your consistency at the end of cooking and then blend.
- Use cooked beef in this recipe unless your soup maker is suitable for raw meat and has a browning function. If it does so add the olive oil, onions, leeks & beef first. Leave to cook for 15 minutes or until the beef is cooked through and then follow the method below.

Add all the ingredients to the soup maker. Cover and leave to cook on medium for 50-60 minutes. Ensure all the ingredients are well combined, tender and piping hot. Blend to your preferred consistency (or leave your machine to do this as programmed). Adjust the seasoning and serve.

This is a great warming soup. Best left chunky and rustic, you could also add some baby sweetcorn and broccoli for even more heartiness.

Mulligatawny Soup
Serves 4

220 CALORIES PER SERVING

Ingredients:

1 tbsp olive oil
75g/3oz lean chicken, beef or pork, finely chopped
1 onion, chopped
2 apples, cored, peeled & chopped
2 celery stalks, chopped

2 tbsp medium curry powder
1 tsp ground coriander/cilantro
500ml/2 cups chicken stock
200g/7oz tinned chopped tomatoes
75g/3oz long grain rice
Salt & pepper to taste

Method:

- Choose your preferred blend function, if required. Otherwise decide on your consistency at the end of cooking and then blend.
- Use cooked meat in this recipe unless your soup maker is suitable for raw meat and has a browning function. If it does so add the olive oil, onions & chopped meat first. Leave to cook for 15 minutes or until the meat is cooked through and then follow the method below.

Add all the ingredients to the soup maker. Cover and leave to cook on high for 30 minutes. Ensure all the ingredients are well combined, tender and piping hot. Blend to your preferred consistency (or leave your machine to do this as programmed). Adjust the seasoning and serve.

It goes without saying that you can adjust the 'heat' of the curry powder in this soup to your preference. Lovely served with Indian naan bread.

Garlic, Bacon & Cannellini Soup
Serves 4

Ingredients:

1 tbsp olive oil
125g/4oz lean back bacon, chopped
4 garlic cloves, crushed
1 onion chopped
1 carrot, chopped
1 celery stalk, chopped
3 tbsp tomato puree/paste

500ml/2 cups vegetable stock
200ml/7oz tinned chopped tomatoes
200g/7oz tinned cannellini beans, drained
1 tsp each dried thyme & oregano
Salt & pepper to taste

Method:

- Choose your preferred blend function, if required. Otherwise decide on your consistency at the end of cooking and then blend.
- Use cooked bacon in this recipe unless your soup maker is suitable for raw meat and has a browning function. If it does so add the olive oil, onions & bacon first. Leave to cook for 5-10 minutes or until the bacon is cooked through and then follow the method below.

Add all the ingredients to the soup maker. Cover and leave to cook on high for 20 minutes. Ensure all the ingredients are well combined, tender and piping hot. Blend to your preferred consistency (or leave your machine to do this as programmed). Adjust the seasoning and serve.

The cannellini beans in this soup can be substituted for any other type of white bean which you prefer, adjust the garlic if you like too.

Spelt Barley & Lamb Soup
Serves 4

290 CALORIES PER SERVING

Ingredients:

1 tbsp olive oil
200g/7oz lean lamb fillet, finely chopped
1 onion, chopped
2 bay leaves (remove before blending)
1 carrot, chopped

1 onion, chopped
50g/2oz spelt barley
2 tbsp freshly chopped flat leaf parsley
750ml/3 cups vegetable stock
Salt & pepper to taste

Method:

- Choose your preferred blend function, if required. Otherwise decide on your consistency at the end of cooking and then blend.
- Use cooked lamb in this recipe unless your soup maker is suitable for raw meat and has a browning function. If it does so add the olive oil, onions & lamb first. Leave to cook for 15 minutes or until the lamb is cooked through and then follow the method below.

Add all the ingredients to the soup maker. Cover and leave to cook on low for 1 ½ -2 hours. Ensure all the ingredients are well combined, tender and piping hot. Blend to your preferred consistency (or leave your machine to do this as programmed). Adjust the seasoning and serve.

Make sure the soup cooks long enough for the lamb to be thoroughly tender. Pearl barley is fine to use for this soup too.

Roast Chicken Soup
Serves 4

295 CALORIES PER SERVING

Ingredients:

1 tbsp olive oil
250g/9oz left-over roast chicken, shredded
750ml/3 cups chicken stock
2 onions, chopped
1 carrot, chopped
1 tbsp thyme leaves, roughly chopped

150g/5oz peas
2 garlic cloves, crushed
4 tbsp fat free Greek yoghurt
1 lemon cut into wedges
Salt & pepper to taste

Method:

- Choose your preferred blend function, if required. Otherwise decide on your consistency at the end of cooking and then blend.
- If your soup maker has a browning function, add the olive oil and onions and leave to cook for a few minutes. Then follow the method below.

Add all the ingredients to the soup maker, except the lemon juice and yoghurt. Cover and leave to cook on high for 30 minutes. Ensure all the ingredients are well combined, tender and piping hot. Blend to your preferred consistency (or leave your machine to do this as programmed). Adjust the seasoning and serve with the lemon wedges and the yoghurt dolloped into each soup bowl.

This is a great way of using up leftover roast chicken. If you don't have enough, supplement with extra breast meat.

Chorizo & Chard Soup

Serves 4

275 CALORIES PER SERVING

Ingredients:

1 tbsp olive oil
175g/6oz chard, trimmed and chopped
2 onions, chopped
4 garlic cloves, crushed
125g/4oz cooking chorizo sausages, sliced

150g/5oz potatoes, peeled & cubed
750ml/3 cups chicken stock
Salt & pepper to taste

Method:

- Choose your preferred blend function, if required. Otherwise decide on your consistency at the end of cooking and then blend.
- Cook the chorizo sausages for this recipe unless your soup maker is suitable for raw meat and has a browning function. If it does so add the olive oil, onions & chorizo first. Leave to cook for 15 minutes or until the chorizo is cooked through and then follow the method below.

Add all the ingredients to the soup maker. Cover and leave to cook on high for 30 minutes. Ensure all the ingredients are well combined, tender and piping hot. Blend to your preferred consistency (or leave your machine to do this as programmed). Adjust the seasoning and serve.

Kale is a great alternative to chard for this recipe, however it can sometimes be a little tough so make sure to trim the thick stalks off.

Sweet Potato & Thai Chicken Soup
Serves 4

290 CALORIES PER SERVING

Ingredients:

1 tbsp olive
200g/7oz skinless chicken breast, chopped
2 garlic cloves, crushed
½ tsp each crushed chilli flakes, ground ginger & fish sauce
2 tbsp red Thai curry paste
750ml/3 cups chicken stock

2 tsp coconut cream
200g/7oz sweet potatoes, peeled & cubed
1 tsp sugar
1 tbsp lime juice
75g/3oz watercress
Salt & pepper to taste

Method:

- Choose your preferred blend function, if required. Otherwise decide on your consistency at the end of cooking and then blend.
- Use cooked chicken in this recipe unless your soup maker is suitable for raw meat and has a browning function. If it does so add the olive oil & chicken first. Leave to cook for 15 minutes or until the chicken is cooked through and then follow the method below.

Add all the ingredients to the soup maker, except the lime juice and watercress. Cover and leave to cook on high for 30 minutes. Ensure all the ingredients are well combined, tender and piping hot. Blend to your preferred consistency (or leave your machine to do this as programmed). Adjust the seasoning, stir through the lime juice and serve with the watercress piled on top of each soup bowl.

The amount of curry paste you use in this recipe can be altered to suit your taste. You can also use green Thai curry paste too.

Porcini & Pancetta Soup

Serves 4

240 CALORIES PER SERVING

Ingredients:

1 tbsp olive oil
75g/3oz cubed pancetta
50g/2oz porcini mushrooms, rehydrated & chopped
50g/2oz chestnut mushrooms, chopped
1 bay leaf (remove before blending)
1 onion, chopped

1 garlic clove, crushed
750ml/3 cups chicken stock
125g/4oz long grain rice
150g/5oz tinned plum tomatoes
1 tbsp freshly chopped flat leaf parsley
Salt & pepper to taste

Method:

- Choose your preferred blend function, if required. Otherwise decide on your consistency at the end of cooking and then blend.
- Use cooked pancetta in this recipe unless your soup maker is suitable for raw meat and has a browning function. If it does so add the olive oil, onions & pancetta first. Leave to cook for 5-10 minutes or until the pancetta is cooked through and then follow the method below.

Add all the ingredients to the soup maker. Cover and leave to cook on high for 30 minutes. Ensure all the ingredients are well combined, tender and piping hot. Remove the bay leaf. Blend to your preferred consistency (or leave your machine to do this as programmed). Adjust the seasoning and serve.

Rehydrate the porcini mushrooms in a little water for half an hour before cooking and use the 'mushroom water' in the soup for additional flavour.

Spiced Turkey & Chickpea Soup
Serves 4

270 CALORIES PER SERVING

Ingredients:

1 tbsp olive oil
250g/9oz lean turkey meat, chopped
1 onion, chopped
1 orange (bell) pepper, deseeded and chopped
1 tsp each ground turmeric & coriander/cilantro
½ tsp crushed chilli flakes

1 tbsp mild curry powder
75g/3oz basmati rice
750ml/3 cups chicken stock
200g/7oz tinned chickpeas, drained
1 tbsp freshly chopped coriander/cilantro
Salt & pepper to taste

Method:

- Choose your preferred blend function, if required. Otherwise decide on your consistency at the end of cooking and then blend.
- Use cooked turkey in this recipe unless your soup maker is suitable for raw meat and has a browning function. If it does so add the olive oil, onions & turkey first. Leave to cook for 15 minutes or until the turkey is cooked through and then follow the method below.

Add all the ingredients to the soup maker, except the chopped coriander. Cover and leave to cook on high for 30 minutes. Ensure all the ingredients are well combined, tender and piping hot. Blend to your preferred consistency (or leave your machine to do this as programmed). Adjust the seasoning, sprinkle with chopped coriander and serve.

This soup is great for using up leftover roast turkey after Christmas or thanksgiving. Feel free to include any leftover cooked vegetables and roast potatoes in the soup too.

71

Lamb & Lentil Soup
Serves 4

270 CALORIES PER SERVING

Ingredients:

1 tbsp olive oil
225g/8oz lean lamb fillet, cubed
500ml/2 cups vegetable stock
250g/9oz fresh tomatoes, chopped
1 onion, chopped

75g/3oz split red lentils
½ tsp each ground turmeric & coriander/cilantro
¼ tsp ground cinnamon
2 tbsp freshly chopped coriander/cilantro
Salt & pepper to taste

Method:

- Choose your preferred blend function, if required. Otherwise decide on your consistency at the end of cooking and then blend.
- Use cooked lamb in this recipe unless your soup maker is suitable for raw meat and has a browning function. If it does so add the olive oil, onions & lamb first. Leave to cook for 15 minutes or until the lamb is cooked through and then follow the method below.

Add all the ingredients to the soup maker, except the chopped coriander. Cover and leave to cook on high for 30 minutes. Ensure all the ingredients are well combined, tender and piping hot. Blend to your preferred consistency (or leave your machine to do this as programmed). Adjust the seasoning, sprinkle with the chopped coriander and serve.

This Moroccan inspired soup is also great with chickpeas and additional cinnamon if you like a really aromatic soup.

German Sausage & Bacon Soup

Serves 4

Ingredients:

1 tbsp olive oil
1 onion, chopped
1 leek, chopped
1 carrot, chopped
1 celery stalk, chopped
175g/6oz lentils
75g/3oz lean back bacon, chopped

175g/6oz frankfurter sausages, sliced
750ml/3 cups chicken stock
1 tbsp freshly chopped parsley
Salt & pepper to taste

Method:

- Choose your preferred blend function, if required. Otherwise decide on your consistency at the end of cooking and then blend.
- Use cooked bacon in this recipe unless your soup maker is suitable for raw meat and has a browning function. If it does so add the olive oil, leek, onions & bacon first. Leave to cook for 5-10 minutes or until the bacon is cooked through and then follow the method below.

Add all the ingredients to the soup maker, except the chopped parsley. Cover and leave to cook on high for 30 minutes. Ensure all the ingredients are well combined, tender and piping hot. Blend to your preferred consistency (or leave your machine to do this as programmed). Adjust the seasoning, sprinkle with the chopped parsley and serve.

Feel free to experiment. If you decide to use a raw sausage instead of frankfurter, ensure your soup maker is able to handle raw meat, otherwise cook before use.

Pork & Rice Soup
Serves 4

215 CALORIES PER SERVING

Ingredients:

1 tbsp olive oil
1 onion, chopped
3 garlic cloves, crushed
1 tsp fish sauce
½ tsp crushed chilli flakes
250g/9oz pork tenderloin,
thinly sliced

100g/3oz long grain rice
750ml/3 cups chicken stock
2 tsp freshly grated ginger
Small bunch spring onions/
scallions, sliced lengthways
Salt & pepper to taste

Method:

- Choose your preferred blend function, if required. Otherwise decide on your consistency at the end of cooking and then blend.
- Use cooked pork in this recipe unless your soup maker is suitable for raw meat and has a browning function. If it does so add the olive oil, onions & pork first. Leave to cook for 15 minutes or until the pork is cooked through and then follow the method below.

Add all the ingredients to the soup maker, except the spring onions. Cover and leave to cook on high for 30 minutes. Ensure all the ingredients are well combined, tender and piping hot. Blend to your preferred consistency (or leave your machine to do this as programmed). Adjust the seasoning, sprinkle with the chopped spring onions and serve.

This soup is also good made with chicken, in fact you can use any leftover lean meat to complement this Spanish inspired dish.

Green Pesto, Tomato & Sausage Soup

Serves 4

Ingredients:

1 tbsp olive oil
350g/12oz lean pork sausages, sliced
1 onion, chopped
1 leek, chopped
75g/3oz red lentils
500ml/2 cups chicken stock

250g/9oz chopped tinned tomatoes
3 tbsp tomato puree
1 tbsp balsamic vinegar
4 tbsp green pesto
Salt & pepper to taste

Method:

- Choose your preferred blend function, if required. Otherwise decide on your consistency at the end of cooking and then blend.
- Use cooked sausages in this recipe unless your soup maker is suitable for raw meat and has a browning function. If it does so add the olive oil, onions, leek & sausages first. Leave to cook for 15 minutes or until the sausages are cooked through and then follow the method below.

Add all the ingredients to the soup maker, except the pesto. Cover and leave to cook on high for 30 minutes. Ensure all the ingredients are well combined, tender and piping hot. Blend to your preferred consistency (or leave your machine to do this as programmed). Adjust the seasoning and serve with a tablespoon of green pesto gently stirred through each bowl soup bowl.

You may need to "balance" the tomatoes in this dish with a little brown sugar. You could also use a spiced sausage if you prefer.

Mixed Bean & Ham Soup

Serves 4

260 CALORIES PER SERVING

Ingredients:

200g/7oz tinned mixed beans
150g/5oz smoked ham, chopped
125g/4oz potatoes, peeled & cubed
1 parsnip, peeled & chopped

750ml/3 cups chicken stock
2 garlic cloves, crushed
125gg/4oz tender stem broccoli, roughly chopped
Salt & pepper to taste

Method:

- Choose your preferred blend function, if required. Otherwise decide on your consistency at the end of cooking and then blend.

Add all the ingredients to the soup maker. Cover and leave to cook on high for 30 minutes. Ensure all the ingredients are well combined, tender and piping hot. Blend to your preferred consistency (or leave your machine to do this as programmed). Adjust the seasoning and serve.

Any kind of cured pork meat will work well in this recipe, try bacon or gammon but be careful with the seasoning as you don't want the soup too salty.

Spicy Sausage & Cabbage Soup

Serves 4

Ingredients:

1 tbsp olive oil
225g/8oz spicy lean sausage, sliced
2 carrots, chopped
1 onion, chopped
1 leek, chopped
75g/3oz potatoes, peeled & cubed

1 green cabbage, chopped
2 garlic cloves, crushed
750ml/3 cups chicken stock
½ tsp crushed chilli flakes
Salt & pepper to taste

Method:

- Choose your preferred blend function, if required. Otherwise decide on your consistency at the end of cooking and then blend.
- Use cooked sausages in this recipe unless your soup maker is suitable for raw meat and has a browning function. If it does so add the olive oil, onions, leek & sausages first. Leave to cook for 15 minutes or until the sausages are cooked through and then follow the method below.

Add all the ingredients to the soup maker. Cover and leave to cook on high for 30 minutes. Ensure all the ingredients are well combined, tender and piping hot. Blend to your preferred consistency (or leave your machine to do this as programmed). Adjust the seasoning and serve.

Add some spinach and additional spice to this dish if you like.

Leek & Back Bacon Soup
Serves 4

290 CALORIES PER SERVING

Ingredients:

1 tbsp olive oil
200g/7oz lean back bacon, chopped
1 onion, chopped
2 leeks, chopped
200g/7oz potatoes, peeled & cubed

1 carrot, chopped
50g/2oz pearl barley
750ml/3 cups chicken stock
Salt & pepper to taste

Method:

- Choose your preferred blend function, if required. Otherwise decide on your consistency at the end of cooking and then blend.
- Use cooked bacon in this recipe unless your soup maker is suitable for raw meat and has a browning function. If it does so add the olive oil, onions & bacon first. Leave to cook for 5-10 minutes or until the bacon is cooked through and then follow the method below.

Add all the ingredients to the soup maker. Cover and leave to cook on high for 30 minutes. Ensure all the ingredients are well combined, tender and piping hot. Blend to your preferred consistency (or leave your machine to do this as programmed). Adjust the seasoning and serve.

Shredded cabbage added to this recipe gives it additional body, plus you could introduced parsnips and/or turnips/swede if you like.

Lamb & Beetroot Soup
Serves 4

180 CALORIES PER SERVING

Ingredients:

1 tbsp olive oil
1 onion, chopped
1 carrot, chopped
1 courgette/zucchini, chopped
175g/6oz lean lamb fillet, chopped
125g/4oz potatoes, peeled & cubed
200g/7oz chopped tinned tomatoes

3 tbsp each tomato puree/ paste & freshly chopped coriander/cilantro
3 garlic cloves chopped
1 tbsp curry powder
500ml/2 cups chicken stock
200g/7oz beetroot, cooked and cubed
1 tsp brown sugar
Salt & pepper to taste

Method:

- Choose your preferred blend function, if required. Otherwise decide on your consistency at the end of cooking and then blend.
- Use cooked lamb in this recipe unless your soup maker is suitable for raw meat and has a browning function. If it does so add the olive oil, onions & lamb first. Leave to cook for 15 minutes or until the lamb is cooked through and then follow the method below.

Add all the ingredients to the soup maker. Cover and leave to cook on high for 30 minutes. Ensure all the ingredients are well combined, tender and piping hot. Blend to your preferred consistency (or leave your machine to do this as programmed). Adjust the seasoning and serve.

Beetroot is a beautiful and sometimes overlooked vegetable. Twinned here with spices and chopped tomatoes it creates a lovely base for the soup.

Skinny Seafood Soups

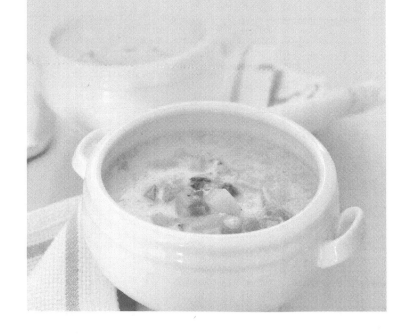

Prawn & Okra Soup
Serves 4

190 CALORIES PER SERVING

Ingredients:

1 tbsp olive oil
125g/4oz cooked peeled prawns
750ml/3 cups fish or vegetable stock
125g/4oz okra, trimmed and sliced
1 onion, chopped
1 bay leaf (remove before blending)

¼ tsp ground all spice
50g/2oz long grain rice
1 tbsp white wine vinegar
1 garlic cloves, crushed
2 tsps anchovy paste
2 tbsp tomato puree/paste
2 slices lean back bacon, chopped
Salt & pepper to taste

Method:

- Choose your preferred blend function, if required. Otherwise decide on your consistency at the end of cooking and then blend.
- Use cooked bacon in this recipe unless your soup maker is suitable for raw meat and has a browning function. If it does so add the olive oil, onions & bacon first. Leave to cook for 5-10 minutes or until the bacon is cooked through and then follow the method below.

Add all the ingredients to the soup maker. Cover and leave to cook on high for 30-40 minutes. Ensure all the ingredients are well combined, tender and piping hot. Remove the bay leaf. Blend to your preferred consistency (or leave your machine to do this as programmed). Adjust the seasoning and serve.

Okra is now available at almost all larger supermarkets. It is used widely in Caribbean cooking and is affectionately known as lady's fingers.

Italian Fish Soup
Serves 4

290 CALORIES PER SERVING

Ingredients:

1 tbsp olive oil
2 onions, chopped
3 garlic cloves, crushed
500ml/2 cups fish or vegetable stock
120ml/½ cup dry white wine
200g/7oz tinned chopped tomatoes
1 tsp each dried thyme,
rosemary & oregano
125g/4oz skinless monkfish fillets, cubed
125g/4oz freshly cooked mussel meat, chopped
125g/4oz cooked peeled prawns
2 tbsp lemon juice
Salt & pepper to taste

Method:

- Ensure your soup maker is suitable for cooking with raw fish. If not you should precook it.
- If your soup maker has a browning function, add the olive oil & onions first. Leave to cook for a few minutes and then follow the method below.

Add all the ingredients to the soup maker, except the lemon juice. Cover and leave to cook on high for 30-40 minutes. Ensure all the ingredients are well combined, tender and piping hot. Adjust the seasoning, stir through the lemon juice and serve.

Use only the freshest cooked mussel meat in this soup recipe.

Coconut Milk & Fresh Crab Soup
Serves 4

145 CALORIES PER SERVING

Ingredients:

1 tbsp olive oil
500ml/2 cups fish or vegetable stock
120ml/ ½ cup coconut cream
1 onion, chopped
2 tbsp fish sauce
2 tbsp red Thai curry paste

300g/11oz cooked fresh white crab meat, shredded
Small bunch spring onions/ scallions, chopped
1 tbsp freshly chopped coriander/cilantro
Salt & pepper to taste

Method:

- Choose your preferred blend function, if required. Otherwise decide on your consistency at the end of cooking and then blend.
- If your soup maker has a browning function, add the olive oil & onions first. Leave to cook for a few minutes and then follow the method below.

Add all the ingredients to the soup maker, except the spring onions and chopped coriander. Cover and leave to cook on high for 30 minutes. Ensure all the ingredients are well combined, tender and piping hot. Blend to your preferred consistency (or leave your machine to do this as programmed). Adjust the seasoning and serve garnished with the chopped coriander and spring onions.

Fresh crab meat is preferable but tinned meat will do fine in this recipe.

Scottish Partan Bree
Serves 4

240
CALORIES
PER SERVING

Ingredients:

1 tbsp olive oil
75g/3oz long grain rice
500ml/2 cups fish or vegetable stock
250ml/1 cup semi skimmed milk

2 tsps anchovy paste
300g/11oz tinned white crab meat
1 tsp lemon juice
2 tbsp freshly chopped chives
Salt & pepper to taste

Method:

- Choose your preferred blend function, if required. Otherwise decide on your consistency at the end of cooking and then blend.

Add all the ingredients to the soup maker, except the lemon juice and chopped chives. Cover and leave to cook on high for 30 minutes. Ensure all the ingredients are well combined, tender and piping hot. Blend to your preferred consistency (or leave your machine to do this as programmed). Stir through the lemon juice, adjust the seasoning and serve with the chives sprinkled over the top.

Otherwise known as Scottish crab bisque, Partan Bree is a North Eastern Scottish speciality which benefits from a swirl of double cream before serving if you have it.

Cullen Skink (Haddock & Potato Soup)

220 CALORIES PER SERVING

Serves 4

Ingredients:

1 tsp butter
1 onion, chopped
1 garlic clove, crushed
500ml/2 cups skimmed milk
350g/12oz fresh mashed potatoes
225g/8oz skinless boneless haddock fillet

2 tbsp freshly chopped flat leaf parsley
1 tbsp lemon juice
2 tbsp crème fraiche
Salt & pepper to taste

Method:

- Ensure your soup maker is suitable for cooking with raw fish. If not you should precook it.
- Choose your preferred blend function, if required. Otherwise decide on your consistency at the end of cooking and then blend.
- If your soup maker has a browning function, add the butter & onions first. Leave to cook for a few minutes and then follow the method below.

Add all the ingredients to the soup maker, except the mash potatoes, lemon juice, crème fraiche and parsley. Cover and leave to cook on medium for 20 minutes. Ensure all the ingredients are well combined, tender and piping hot. Blend to your preferred consistency (or leave your machine to do this as programmed). Add the mashed potatoes, stir and warm through for a few minutes. Stir through the crème fraiche and lemon juice, adjust the seasoning and serve with the parsley sprinkled on top.

Dyed smoked haddock is traditionally used in this Scottish recipe but undyed haddock will taste just as good.

Thai Fish & Pak Choi Soup

Serves 4

290
CALORIES
PER SERVING

Ingredients:

125g/4oz egg noodles
750ml/3cups chicken or fish stock
200g/7oz skinless, boneless haddock fillets
1 red (bell) pepper, deseeded and sliced
2 tbsp Thai red curry paste

2 tbsp fish sauce
1 tbsp sweet chilli sauce
125g/4oz cooked peeled prawns
1 pak choi, chopped
2 tbsp freshly chopped coriander/cilantro

Method:

- Ensure your soup maker is suitable for cooking with raw fish. If not you should precook it.
- Choose your preferred blend function, if required. Otherwise decide on your consistency at the end of cooking and then blend.

Add all the ingredients to the soup maker, except the chopped coriander. Cover and leave to cook on high for 30 minutes. Ensure all the ingredients are well combined, tender and piping hot. Blend to your preferred consistency (or leave your machine to do this as programmed). Adjust the seasoning and serve with the chopped coriander sprinkled over the top.

Any kind of noodles are fine in this dish. You could also reserve some of the pak choi leaves and sprinkle over as a finely chopped garnish after serving if you want a little crunch.

Cod & Broccoli Soup
Serves 4

290 CALORIES PER SERVING

Ingredients:

1 tsp olive oil

200g/7oz skinless boneless cod fillet

125g/4oz potatoes, peeled & chopped

250ml/1 cups semi skimmed milk

500ml/2 cups fish or vegetable stock

125g/4oz tender stem broccoli, roughly chopped

75g/3oz sweetcorn

1 lemon cut into wedges

Small bunch spring onions/ scallions, thinly sliced lengthways

Salt & pepper to taste

Method:

- Ensure your soup maker is suitable for cooking with raw fish. If not you should precook it.
- Choose your preferred blend function, if required. Otherwise decide on your consistency at the end of cooking and then blend.

Add all the ingredients to the soup maker, except the spring onions and lemon wedges. Cover and leave to cook on medium for 30-40 minutes. Ensure all the ingredients are well combined, tender and piping hot. Blend to your preferred consistency (or leave your machine to do this as programmed). Adjust the seasoning and serve with lemon wedges and the chopped spring onions sprinkled over the top.

Any firm meaty white fish will do well in this recipe. Try to use purple sprouting broccoli if you can as it's super tender and naturally sweet when in season.

Garlic Mussels & Plum Tomato Soup

Serves 4

Ingredients:

1 tbsp olive oil
5 garlic cloves, crushed
200g/7oz cooked mussel meat
(out of their shells), chopped
1 large bunch basil leaves,
chopped
4 sweet shallots, chopped

200g/7oz fresh plum tomatoes
1 tbsp tomato puree/paste
500ml/2 cups fish or vegetable
stock
120ml/ ½ cup dry white wine
Salt & pepper to taste

Method:

- Choose your preferred blend function, if required. Otherwise decide on your consistency at the end of cooking and then blend.

Add all the ingredients to the soup maker. Cover and leave to cook on high for 40 minutes. Ensure all the ingredients are well combined, tender and piping hot. Blend to your preferred consistency (or leave your machine to do this as programmed). Adjust the seasoning and serve.

Any ripe tomatoes works well in this recipe. Add a little brown sugar if you need to balance the acidity in this dish.

Creamy Salmon & Watercress Soup

Serves 4

Ingredients:

1 tsp butter
200g/7oz boneless, skinless salmon fillet, cooked and flaked
1 onion, chopped
1 leek, chopped
125g/4oz potatoes, peeled & cubed

500ml/2 cups fish stock
120ml/ ½ cup semi skimmed milk
120ml/ ½ cup single cream
75g/3oz watercress
Salt & pepper to taste

Method:

- Choose your preferred blend function, if required. Otherwise decide on your consistency at the end of cooking and then blend.

Add all the ingredients to the soup maker, except the salmon, milk, cream and watercress. Cover and leave to cook on medium for 30 minutes. Ensure all the ingredients are well combined, tender and piping hot. Blend to your preferred consistency (or leave your machine to do this as programmed). Add the cream, milk, salmon & watercress and warm thoroughly for a few minutes. Adjust the seasoning and serve.

You could alter this recipe to use smoked salmon instead. Chop the smoked salmon and add just before serving.

Tomato, Saffron & Seafood Soup

210 CALORIES PER SERVING

Serves 4

Ingredients:

1 tbsp olive oil
3 garlic cloves, crushed
1 onion, chopped
Half a fennel bulb, chopped
250g/9oz skinless, boneless turbot fillet, chopped
125g/4oz shelled cooked prawns
Large pinch saffron threads

½ tsp crushed chilli flakes
750ml/3 cups chicken stock
1 fresh tomato, chopped
3 tbsp each tomato puree/ paste & freshly chopped flat leaf parsley
Zest of 1 orange
Salt & pepper to taste

Method:

- Ensure your soup maker is suitable for cooking with raw fish. If not you should precook it.
- Choose your preferred blend function, if required. Otherwise decide on your consistency at the end of cooking and then blend.
- If your soup maker has a browning function, add the olive oil & onions first. Leave to cook for a few minutes and then follow the method below.

Add all the ingredients to the soup maker, except the parsley. Cover and leave to cook on high for 30 minutes. Ensure all the ingredients are well combined, tender and piping hot. Blend to your preferred consistency (or leave your machine to do this as programmed). Adjust the seasoning and serve with chopped parsley sprinkled over the top.

Turbot is good in this soup but any other meaty white fish will do as well. Don't chop the fish too small, instead leave it in reasonably large chunks.

Indian Prawn Soup
Serves 4

290 CALORIES PER SERVING

Ingredients:

1 tbsp olive oil
2 garlic cloves, crushed
200g/7oz peeled cooked prawns
1 onion, chopped
75g/3oz basmati rice
2 fresh tomatoes, chopped

750ml/3 cups fish stock
1 tsp each ground turmeric, cumin, chilli powder & coriander/cilantro
2 tbsp coconut cream
Salt & pepper to taste

Method:

- Choose your preferred blend function, if required. Otherwise decide on your consistency at the end of cooking and then blend.
- If your soup maker has a browning function, add the olive oil & onions first. Leave to cook for a few minutes and then follow the method below.

Add all the ingredients to the soup maker. Cover and leave to cook on high for 20 minutes. Ensure all the ingredients are well combined, tender and piping hot. Adjust the seasoning and serve.

The basmati rice gives this soup a really robust base. To make it a main-course meal serve with some garlic naan bread.

Liguria Fish Soup
Serves 4

Ingredients:

1 tbsp olive oil
250g/9oz boneless skinless firm white fish fillets
1 onion, chopped
1 carrot, chopped
1 tsp anchovy paste
1 celery stalk, chopped
500ml/2 cups fish or chicken stock

250ml/1 cup dry white wine
3 garlic cloves, crushed
1 tomato, chopped
3 tbsp freshly chopped flat leaf parsley
Salt & pepper to taste

Method:

- Ensure your soup maker is suitable for cooking with raw fish. If not you should precook it.
- Choose your preferred blend function, if required. Otherwise decide on your consistency at the end of cooking and then blend.
- If your soup maker has a browning function, add the olive oil & onions first. Leave to cook for a few minutes and then follow the method below.

Add all the ingredients to the soup maker, except the chopped parsley. Cover and leave to cook on high for 30 minutes. Ensure all the ingredients are well combined, tender and piping hot. Blend to your preferred consistency (or leave your machine to do this as programmed). Adjust the seasoning and serve with chopped parsley sprinkled over the top.

Originating from the Italian costal region of Liguria, this soup is best served pureed to a completely smooth texture and eaten with slices of fresh crusty bread.

Skinny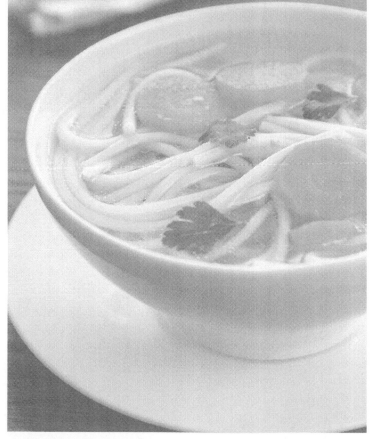
Ramen, Noodle
& Laksa Soups

Thai Tofu & Noodle Soup

Serves 4

195 CALORIES PER SERVING

Ingredients:

1 tbsp olive oil
1 onion, chopped
2 sticks lemongrass, bashed
(remove before blending)
2 tsp freshly grated ginger
4 garlic cloves, crushed
750ml/3cups vegetable stock
225g/8oz tofu, cubed

1 tbsp each freshly chopped
mint & coriander/cilantro
2 tbsp fish sauce
2 tbsp sweet chilli sauce
1 tsp brown sugar
400g/14oz cooked egg noodles
Salt & pepper to taste

Method:

- This soup does not require blending.
- If your soup maker has a browning function, add the olive oil and onions first and leave to brown for a few minutes.

Add all the ingredients to the soup maker, except the noodles. Cover and leave to cook on high for 20 minutes. Ensure all the ingredients are well combined, tender and piping hot. Add the cooked noodles to each soup bowl. Adjust the seasoning and serve.

This lovely noodle dish can be stretched with some finely shredded carrots, pak choi and bean sprouts after cooking to add a fresh crunch.

Ramen Pork Soup
Serves 4

298
CALORIES
PER SERVING

Ingredients:

1 tsp vegetable oil
225g/8oz ramen noodles
250g/9oz pork tenderloin, chopped
750ml/3cups chicken stock
Large bunch spring onions/scallions, chopped
1 tbsp freshly grated ginger

225g/8oz ready to use bamboo shoots
2 tbsp soy sauce
1 tbsp rice wine vinegar
1 tsp brown sugar
75g/3oz spinach, chopped
Salt & pepper to taste

Method:

- This soup does not require blending.
- Use cooked pork in this recipe unless your soup maker is suitable for raw meat and has a browning function. If it does, add the pork first and leave to cook for 15 minutes or until the pork is cooked through and then follow the method below.

Add all the ingredients to the soup maker. Cover and leave to cook on high for 20 minutes. Ensure all the ingredients are well combined, tender and piping hot. Adjust the seasoning and serve.

Ramen has become a widely eaten dish in the west over recent years as a result of the popularity of fast food Japanese noodle restaurants.

Shiitake & Onion Noodle Soup
Serves 4

185 CALORIES PER SERVING

Ingredients:

1 tbsp olive oil
150g/5oz fine egg noodles
125g/4oz shiitake mushrooms, pre soaked and chopped
1 tsp each ground turmeric & garlic powder
1 tsp crushed chilli flakes

1 tbsp freshly grated ginger
1 tsp brown sugar
750ml/3cups chicken stock
2 tsp shrimp paste
1 regular white onion, chopped
1 red onion, cut into rings
Salt & pepper to taste

Method:

- This soup does not require blending.
- If your soup maker has a browning function, add the olive oil and white onion first and leave to brown for a few minutes.

Add all the ingredients to the soup maker, except the sliced red onion. Cover and leave to cook on high for 20 minutes. Ensure all the ingredients are well combined, tender and piping hot. Adjust the seasoning and serve with the sliced red onions arranged on top of each bowl of soup.

Leaving the red onions raw gives this dish a lovely fresh crunch. You could also add a twist of lime to freshen it even further.

Mullet & Lemongrass Laksa

Serves 4

275 CALORIES PER SERVING

Ingredients:

450g/1lb skinless, boneless mullet fillet
750ml/3cups fish or chicken stock
1 onion, chopped
1 tbsp tamarind paste
1 tsp caster sugar
1 tbsp fish sauce

225g/8oz rice noodles
1 stalk fresh lemon grass, peeled and finely chopped
3 garlic cloves, crushed
75g/3oz bean sprouts
Large bunch fresh basil, chopped

Method:

- This soup does not require blending.
- Ensure your soup maker is suitable for cooking with raw fish. If not you should pre-cook it.

Add all the ingredients to the soup maker, except the bean sprouts. Cover and leave to cook on high for 20 minutes. Ensure all the ingredients are well combined, tender and piping hot. Adjust the seasoning and serve with bean sprouts piled on top of each bowl of soup.

Chopped peanuts sprinkled over the top of the noodle soup makes a lovely additional garnish to this dish.

Spiced Prawn Vermicelli Soup
Serves 4

Ingredients:

125g/4oz vermicelli noodles
200g/7oz cooked peeled
prawns, chopped
750ml/3 cups fish or chicken
stock
2 tbsp coconut cream
2 tbsp fish sauce
½ tsp cayenne pepper
1 red chilli, deseeded and finely
chopped
1 tsp shrimp paste
3 garlic cloves crushed
1 tsp each ground turmeric &
coriander/cilantro
2 tsp freshly grated ginger
1 fresh lemon grass stalk,
peeled & finely chopped
Salt & pepper to taste

Method:

- This soup does not require blending.

Add all the ingredients to the soup maker, except the coconut cream. Cover and leave to cook on high for 20 minutes. Ensure all the ingredients are well combined, tender and piping hot. Stir in the coconut cream and warm through for a minute or two. Adjust the seasoning and serve.

Stirring the coconut cream through after cooking means there is no chance it will 'split' during cooking and spoil the soup.

Moroccan Chicken Noodle Soup

Serves 4

Ingredients:

1 tbsp olive oil
350g/12oz skinless chicken breast, cubed
1 onion, chopped
150g/5oz fine egg noodles
1 carrot, chopped
125g/4oz sweet potato, peeled & chopped

1 tsp each paprika, ground cinnamon & coriander/cilantro
½ tsp ground nutmeg
750ml/3cups chicken stock
3 tbsp freshly chopped flat leaf parsley
Salt & pepper to taste

Method:

- This soup does not require blending
- Use cooked chicken in this recipe unless your soup maker is suitable for raw meat and has a browning function. If it does so add the olive oil, onions & chicken first. Leave to cook for 15 minutes or until the chicken is cooked through and then follow the method below.

Add all the ingredients to the soup maker except the parsley. Cover and leave to cook on high for 20 minutes. Ensure all the ingredients are well combined, tender and piping hot. Adjust the seasoning and serve with parsley sprinkled on top.

A pinch of saffron in this dish also adds to the Moroccan fragrance which will fill your kitchen when you cook this soup.

Spicy Chicken & Egg Noodle Soup

295 CALORIES PER SERVING

Serves 4

Ingredients:

1 tbsp olive oil
450g/1lb skinless chicken breast, cubed
150g/5oz fine egg noodles
1 onion chopped
5 shallots, chopped
750ml/3cups chicken stock
4 free range eggs, hardboiled, peeled & halved
1 tbsp freshly grated ginger

1 tsp each ground coriander/cilantro, turmeric & crushed chilli flakes
1 tbsp freshly chopped coriander/cilantro
2 stalks lemongrass, peeled & finely chopped
125g/4oz beansprouts
2 tbsp lime juice
Salt & pepper to taste

Method:

- This soup does not require blending
- Use cooked chicken in this recipe unless your soup maker is suitable for raw meat and has a browning function. If it does so add the olive oil, onions, shallots & chicken first. Leave to cook for 15 minutes or until the chicken is cooked through and then follow the method below.

Add all the ingredients to the soup maker except the lime juice, bean sprouts and hard boiled eggs. Cover and leave to cook on high for 20 minutes. Ensure all the ingredients are well combined, tender and piping hot. Adjust the seasoning, stir in the lime and serve with the bean sprouts and two egg halves on top.

Lemongrass can be an acquired taste, if you are a fan of the taste increase the quantity of chopped fresh lemongrass in the recipe.

Chicken & Cabbage Ramen Soup
Serves 4

240
CALORIES
PER SERVING

Ingredients:

1 tsp vegetable oil
225g/8oz ramen noodles
1 onion, chopped
250g/9oz skinless chicken breast, cubed
750ml/3cups chicken stock
1 tbsp freshly grated ginger
125g/4oz baby corn
125g/4oz ready to use bamboo shoots
1 small pointed cabbage, chopped
2 tbsp soy sauce
1 tbsp fish sauce
1 tbsp rice wine vinegar
1 tsp brown sugar
Salt & pepper to taste

Method:

- This soup does not require blending.
- Use cooked chicken in this recipe unless your soup maker is suitable for raw meat and has a browning function. If it does, add the olive oil, onion and chicken first. Leave to cook for 15 minutes or until the chicken is cooked through and then follow the method below.

Add all the ingredients to the soup maker. Cover and leave to cook on high for 20 minutes. Ensure all the ingredients are well combined, tender and piping hot. Adjust the seasoning and serve.

Use Chinese cabbage if you can and serve with rice crackers.

Skinny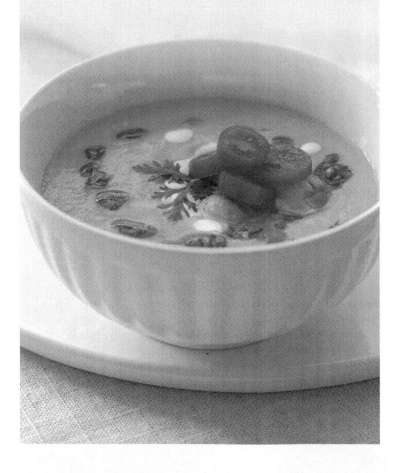
Chilled Soups

Lettuce & Crème Fraiche Soup
Serves 4

Ingredients:

1 tbsp olive oil
2 cucumbers, peeled & chopped
1 romaine lettuce, shredded
1 leek, chopped
1 onion, chopped

125g/4oz potatoes, peeled & cubed
750ml/3cups vegetable stock
120ml/ ½ cup crème fraiche
2 tbsp chopped chives
Salt & pepper to taste

Method:

- Choose your preferred blend function, if required. Otherwise decide on your consistency at the end of cooking and then blend.
- If your soup maker has a browning function, add the olive oil, onions and leeks first and leave to brown for a few minutes.

Add all the ingredients to the soup maker, except half the shredded lettuce, all the crème fraiche and the chopped chives. Cover and leave to cook on high for 20 minutes. Ensure all the ingredients are well combined, tender and piping hot. Blend to your preferred consistency (or leave your machine to do this as programmed). Add the reserved shredded lettuce and leave to warm through for a further 2-3 minutes. Leave to cool. Chill, adjust the seasoning, add a dollop of crème fraiche to each bowl, stir through, garnish with chopped chives and serve.

This light delicate soup is delicious for the summer months when you want a quick and tasty light meal.

Chunky Spanish Gazpacho
Serves 4

148 CALORIES PER SERVING

Ingredients:

1 tbsp olive oil
2 garlic cloves, crushed
1kg/2lb 4oz vine ripened
tomatoes
2 red peppers, chopped

1 onion, chopped
2 tbsp balsamic vinegar
1 tsp brown sugar
Salt & pepper to taste

Method:

- Choose your preferred blend function, if required. Otherwise decide on your consistency at the end of cooking and then blend.
- If your soup maker has a browning function, add the olive oil and onions first and leave to brown for a few minutes.

Add all the ingredients to the soup maker. Cover and leave to cook on high for 30 minutes. Ensure all the ingredients are well combined, tender and piping hot. Blend to your preferred consistency (or leave your machine to do this as programmed). Leave to cool. Chill, adjust the seasoning and serve.

This traditional Spanish soup is best served chunky. Chopped fresh basil would add a lovely garnish as would some rustic homemade croutons.

Lemon & Avocado Soup

Serves 4

280 CALORIES PER SERVING

Ingredients:

1 tsp olive oil
2 tsp lemon juice
1 onion, chopped
500ml/2 cups vegetable stock
2 ripe avocadoes, flesh scooped out
1 large cucumber, peeled & chopped

60ml/ ¼ cup whole milk
60ml/ ¼ cup skimmed milk
1 vine ripened tomato, chopped
Salt & pepper to taste

Method:

- Choose your preferred blend function, if required. Otherwise decide on your consistency at the end of cooking and then blend.
- If your soup maker has a browning function, add the olive oil and onions first and leave to brown for a few minutes.

Add all the ingredients to the soup maker, except the chopped tomato and half the chopped cucumber. Cover and leave to cook on high for 10 minutes. Ensure all the ingredients are well combined, tender and piping hot. Blend to your preferred consistency (or leave your machine to do this as programmed). Leave to cool. Chill, adjust the seasoning and serve with the reserved chopped tomatoes and cucumber sprinkled over each bowl.

The avocados provide a lovely rich base for this soup which is super creamy.

Minted Yoghurt & Chilled Cucumber Soup
Serves 4

298
CALORIES
PER SERVING

Ingredients:

1 large cucumber, peeled & diced
1 garlic clove, chopped
½ tsp cayenne pepper
250ml/1 cup tomato juice

250ml/1 cup fat free Greek yoghurt
250ml/1 cup cooled chicken stock
2 tbsp freshly chopped mint
Salt & pepper to taste

Method:

Add all the ingredients to the soup maker. Cover, blend until smooth and leave to cool. Chill, adjust the seasoning and serve.

This chilled soup requires no cooking. Additional chopped mint leaves add a great garnish, plus a dash of double cream is delicious.

Melon & Fresh Ginger Soup
Serves 4

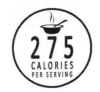

275 CALORIES PER SERVING

Ingredients:

500g/1lb 2oz cantaloupe melon
flesh, chopped
1 tbsp freshly grated ginger
500ml/2 cups fat free Greek
yoghurt

1 tbsp brown sugar
250ml/1 cup single cream
1 tsp freshly chopped mint
Salt & pepper to taste

Method:

Add all the ingredients to the soup maker. Cover and blend until smooth. Chill, adjust the seasoning and serve.

Another 'no cook' soup, the ginger quantity can be altered to reflect your preference. Add a little more sugar if the melon is not ripe enough.

Chilled Almond Soup
Serves 4

185 CALORIES PER SERVING

Ingredients:

1 tbsp extra virgin olive oil
200g/7oz whole blanched
almonds, chopped
2 garlic cloves, crushed
1 tbsp balsamic vinegar
1 tsp salt

2 cups crushed ice
2 cups/500ml water
125g/4oz seedless grapes
1 apple, peeled & cored
Salt & pepper to taste

Method:

Add all the ingredients to the soup maker, except the ice cubes.
Cover and blend until smooth. Chill, adjust the seasoning and
serve with the crushed ice in each bowl.

*The almonds are best bought unprocessed and
blanched at home by covering in boiling water for 4
minutes and then squeezing out of their skins.*

Chilled Lemongrass & Fresh Coriander Soup

190 CALORIES PER SERVING

Serves 4

Ingredients:

1 tbsp olive oil
3 fresh lemongrass stems, stripped and finely chopped
3 tbsp freshly chopped coriander/cilantro
2 onions, chopped

250g/9oz potatoes, peeled & cubed
500ml/2 cups chicken stock
250ml/1 cup milk
1 lemon cut into wedges
Salt & pepper to taste

Method:

- Choose your preferred blend function, if required. Otherwise decide on your consistency at the end of cooking and then blend.
- If your soup maker has a browning function, add the olive oil and onions first and leave to brown for a few minutes.

Add all the ingredients to the soup maker, except the lemon wedges and milk. Cover and leave to cook on high for 30 minutes. Ensure all the ingredients are well combined, tender and piping hot. Blend to your preferred consistency (or leave your machine to do this as programmed). Add the milk and leave to cool. Chill, adjust the seasoning and serve with lemon wedges on the side.

Fresh lemongrass is widely available now at most Asian supermarkets and adds an unusual flavour to this lovely light soup recipe.

Chilled Zucchini & Cream Soup

Serves 4

220 CALORIES PER SERVING

Ingredients:

1 tbsp olive oil
2 onions, chopped
450g/1lb courgettes/zucchini, chopped

500 ml/2 cups vegetable stock
2 tbsp freshly chopped mint
250ml/1 cup single cream
Salt & pepper to taste

Method:

- Choose your preferred blend function, if required. Otherwise decide on your consistency at the end of cooking and then blend.
- If your soup maker has a browning function, add the olive oil and onions first and leave to brown for a few minutes.

Add all the ingredients to the soup maker, except the cream. Cover and leave to cook on high for 30 minutes. Ensure all the ingredients are well combined, tender and piping hot. Blend to your preferred consistency (or leave your machine to do this as programmed). Leave to cool. Chill, stir through the cream, adjust the seasoning and serve.

This soup is best eaten in the summer when courgettes are in season and plentiful. You could also add some freshly chopped basil during cooking or as a garnish.

Elegant Asparagus Soup

Serves 4

Ingredients:

1 tbsp olive oil
300g/11oz fresh asparagus spears, trimmed and chopped
1 onion, chopped
200g/7oz potatoes, peeled & cubed

500ml/2 cups chicken stock
120ml/ ½ cup single cream
Salt & pepper to taste

Method:

- Choose your preferred blend function, if required. Otherwise decide on your consistency at the end of cooking and then blend.
- If your soup maker has a browning function, add the olive oil and onions first and leave to brown for a few minutes.

Add all the ingredients to the soup maker, except the cream. Cover and leave to cook on high for 30 minutes. Ensure all the ingredients are well combined, tender and piping hot. Blend to your preferred consistency (or leave your machine to do this as programmed). Leave to cool. Chill, stir through the cream, adjust the seasoning and serve.

Asparagus spears are some of the most delicious of all seasonal offerings. Using as soon as possible after harvesting makes the most of their natural sweetness.

Beetroot & Dill Soup
Serves 4

120 CALORIES PER SERVING

Ingredients:

1 tbsp olive oil
400g/14oz cooked beetroot
125g/4oz shallots, chopped
2 bay leaves (removed before blending)
1 tsp freshly chopped thyme

1 tbsp freshly chopped dill
3 garlic cloves, crushed
1 carrot, chopped
750ml/3cups vegetable stock
4 tbsp sour cream
Salt and pepper to taste

Method:

- Choose your preferred blend function, if required. Otherwise decide on your consistency at the end of cooking and then blend.
- If your soup maker has a browning function, add the olive oil and onions first and leave to brown for a few minutes.

Add all the ingredients to the soup maker, except the sour cream and half the chopped dill. Cover and leave to cook on high for 30 minutes. Ensure all the ingredients are well combined, tender and piping hot. Remove the bay leaf and blend to your preferred consistency (or leave your machine to do this as programmed). Leave to cool. Chill, stir through the sour cream, adjust the seasoning, sprinkle with the reserved dill and serve.

The beetroot is this recipe can be roasted or boiled before using in the soup - either will work well really well.

Conversion Chart
Weights for dry ingredients:

Metric	Imperial
7g	¼ oz
15g	½ oz
20g	¾ oz
25g	1 oz
40g	1½oz
50g	2oz
60g	2½oz
75g	3oz
100g	3½oz
125g	4oz
140g	4½oz
150g	5oz
165g	5½oz
175g	6oz
200g	7oz
225g	8oz
250g	9oz
275g	10oz
300g	11oz
350g	12oz
375g	13oz
400g	14oz
425g	15oz
450g	1lb
500g	1lb 2oz
550g	1¼lb
600g	1lb 5oz
650g	1lb 7oz
675g	1½lb
700g	1lb 9oz
750g	1lb 11oz
800g	1¾lb
900g	2lb
1kg	2¼lb
1.1kg	2½lb
1.25kg	2¾lb
1.35kg	3lb
1.5kg	3lb 6oz
1.8kg	4lb
2kg	4½lb
2.25kg	5lb
2.5kg	5½lb
2.75kg	6lb

Conversion Chart

Liquid measures:

Metric	Imperial	Aus	US
25ml	1fl oz		
60ml	2fl oz	¼ cup	¼ cup
75ml	3fl oz		
100ml	3½fl oz		
120ml	4fl oz	½ cup	½ cup
150ml	5fl oz		
175ml	6fl oz	¾ cup	¾ cup
200ml	7fl oz		
250ml	8fl oz	1 cup	1 cup
300ml	10fl oz/½ pt	1¼ cups	
360ml	12fl oz		
400ml	14fl oz		
450ml	15fl oz	2 cups	2 cups/1 pint
600ml	1 pint	1 pint	2½ cups
750ml	1¼ pint		
900ml	1½ pints		
1 litre	1½ pints	1¾ pints	1 quart

Other CookNation Titles

You may also be interested in other titles in the CookNation series

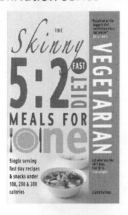

The Skinny 5:2 Fast Diet Vegetarian Meals For One
Single Serving Fast Day Recipes & Snacks Under 100, 200 & 300 Calories.

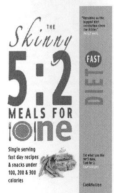

The Skinny 5:2 Fast Diet Meals For One
Single Serving Fast Day Recipes & Snacks Under 100, 200 & 300 Calories.

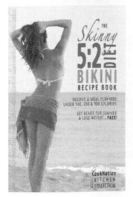

The Skinny 5:2 Bikini Diet Recipe Book
Recipes & Meal Planners Under 100, 200 & 300 Calories. Get Ready For Summer & Lose Weight... FAST!

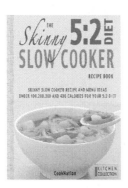

The Skinny 5:2 Slow Cooker Recipe Book
Skinny Slow Cooker Recipe And Menu Ideas Under 100, 200, 300 & 400 Calories For Your 5:2 Diet.

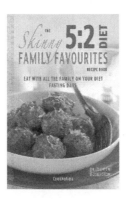

The Skinny 5:2 Family Favourites Recipe Book
(UK Edition)
Eat With All the Family On Your Diet Fasting Days

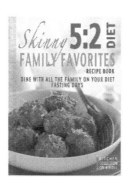

The Skinny 5:2 Family Favorites Recipe Book
(USA Edition)
Dine With All The Family On Your Diet Fasting Days

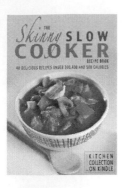

**The Skinny Slow Cooker
Recipe Book**
40 Delicious Recipes Under
300, 400 And 500 Calories.

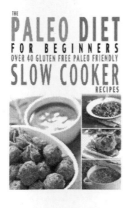

**The Paleo Diet For
Beginners Slow Cooker
Recipe Book**
Over 40 Gluten Free Paleo
Friendly Slow Cooker
Recipes.

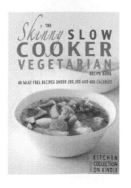

**The Skinny Slow Cooker
Vegetarian Recipe Book**
40 Delicious Recipes Under
200, 300 And 400 Calories.

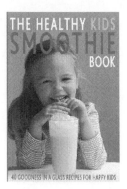

The Healthy Kids Smoothie Book
40 Delicious Goodness In A Glass Recipes for Happy Kids.

Find all these great titles by searching under '**CookNation**' on Amazon.

Review

If you enjoyed The Skinny Soup Maker Recipe Book we'd really appreciate your feedback. Reviews help others decide if this is the right book for them so a moment of your time would be appreciated. Thank you.